COOKING WITH SEA VEGETABLES

An invaluable introduction to the use of sea vegetables in cooking, containing a wealth of delicious and nutritious recipes.

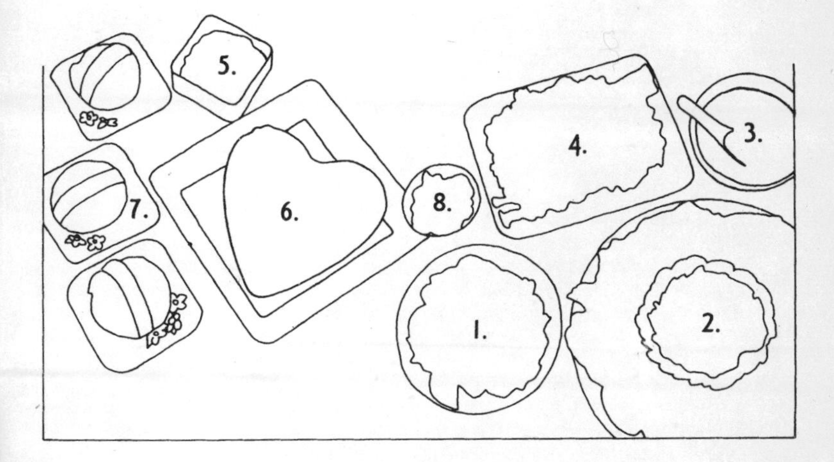

Illustrated on cover:

1. Dressed Salad with Wakame (page 87)
2. Dulse Cocktail (page 97)
3. Dressing for Dulse Cocktail (page 97)
4. Arame with Broccoli and Mushrooms (page 119)
5. Agar-Agar Flakes (page 120)
6. Strawberry Kanten (page 127)
7. Tangerine Kanten (page 129)
8. Dried Carragheen (page 131)

COOKING WITH SEA VEGETABLES

A collection of naturally delicious dishes using to the full the bountiful harvest of the oceans

Peter and Montse Bradford

Illustrated by Sue Reid

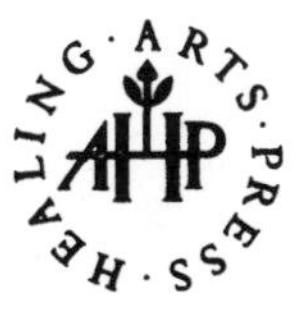

HEALING ARTS PRESS
ROCHESTER, VERMONT

Healing Arts Press
One Park Street
Rochester, Vermont 05767
www.innertraditions.com

Copyright © 1985, 1988 by Peter and Montse Bradford

All rights reserved. No part of this book may be reproduced or utilized in any form or by any means, electronic or mechanical, including photocopying, recording, or by any information storage and retrieval system, without permission in writing from the publisher.

Note to the reader: This book is intended as an informational guide. The remedies, approaches, and techniques described herein are meant to supplement, and not to be a substitute for, professional medical care or treatment. They should not be used to treat a serious ailment without prior consultation with a qualified healthcare professional.

LIBRARY OF CONGRESS CATALOGING-IN-PUBLICATION DATA

Bradford, Peter, 1944–
Cooking with sea vegetables.
Reprint. Originally published: New York: Thorsons Publishers, 1985.
Bibliography: p.
Includes index.
1. Marine algae as food. 2. Cookery (Marine algae).
I. Bradford, Montse. II. Title.
TX402.B73 1988 641.6 88–32002
ISBN 0-89281-283-4

Printed and bound in India

15 14 13 12 11 10 9 8 7 6

Healing Arts Press is a division of Inner Traditions International

Acknowledgements

We would like to acknowledge our teachers and friends in our venture of discovering sea vegetables. To Georges and Lima Ohsawa, Michio and Aveline Kushi, Herman and Cornelia Aihara, Denny and Judy Waxman, Bill Tara and Susan Stokes, we offer our thanks. Without their inspiration we would not have been able to write this book. We would also like to thank our suppliers, both in Japan and in the West, for their efforts in making sea vegetables available in our local stores.

Contents

Introduction

The purpose of this book is to provide a simple practical introduction to the use of sea vegetables in daily cooking. Traditionally, sea vegetables have been used by many societies throughout the world. Only recently in some areas has their use become eclipsed by modern factory-produced foods. Even so, almost everyone is still consuming sea plants in some form or other. The head on a glass of beer, or the texture of an ice cream is dependent on the use of sea vegetable extracts. Now there is a revival, though, in the traditional use of these plants, as whole natural foods in their own right. Our recipes follow this tradition, using sea vegetables in natural cookery without any animal or dairy products, without any sugar or refined ingredients and, of course, without any chemical additives or preservatives.

We prefer the term *sea vegetable*, rather than *seaweed*. To our understanding, a weed is a plant that is either growing where it is not wanted, or for which there is no practical use. Both descriptions, in our experience, are inaccurate. We have been using sea vegetables in our daily meals for many years now, and have become familiar with the wide range that is available. The aroma of the sea shore is often the smell of decay from washed-up dying sea plants. But freshly harvested live sea plants, carefully dried and cooked with care, are as varied and useful as their cousins on the land. And contrary to popular belief, they are tasty and in our opinion, an essential ingredient in preparing balanced nutritious meals. In this book we would like to share some of our discoveries of the exciting dishes that can be prepared using these 'vegetables from the sea'. They range from soups to starters, through entrées, side dishes, salads, pickles and condiments, to desserts and snacks.

Today the Japanese industry dominates the world market of sea vegetables, and is currently our major source of supply. For this reason throughout the book we primarily use the Japanese names as they are better known than the botanical or local names. At the end of the book we have included a chart that cross-references the local and botanical names for all the common sea vegetables.

The Delights of Sea Vegetables

Not Just a Modern Fad

Since ancient times people all over the world living near the sea have incorporated sea vegetables in their daily meals. Even remote from the oceans, water algae from lakes and rivers have regularly been used as food. In China in the sixth century B.C., Sze Tsu wrote that, 'sea vegetables are a delicacy fit for the most honoured guest'. Over two thousand years ago the ancient Koreans were sending sea vegetables to the Imperial Court of China, where they were prized for their medicinal value. At that time the *Ehr Ya* Chinese encyclopaedia records twelve species in regular use.

Throughout the Pacific Islands sea vegetables have a long history of use. The ancient kings of Hawaii cultivated or harvested over seventy varieties of *limu* around their coastline. The Maoris of New Zealand have long used *karengo*, a kind of nori, in soups and salads. During the second world war Maori soldiers sustained themselves on *karengo* during their long marches through the arid Middle East.

There is a well recorded use of sea vegetables in north west Europe as well. The ancient Celts and Vikings chewed dulse on their travels. Wild nori, *laver* (Latin for 'water plant'), has been popular since Roman times and *laverbread* is still sold today in the markets of south Wales. *Bladderwrack*, *carragheen*, *dabberlocks*, *sea lettuce*, *sloke*, *tangle* and *samphire* are also still remembered as food in various parts of the British Isles.

The Japanese, perhaps more than anyone, with their long indented coastline, have most developed the culinary potential of sea vegetables. All the major varieties currently consumed were registered as part of the annual tribute to the court by the eighth century AD. So popular have sea vegetables become in Japan that in recent times demand has outstripped the natural wild supply of several species and these are now widely cultivated around the coastline. On visits to Japan we have seen some coastal waters as intensively 'farmed' as the land itself. Current production of nori alone is a staggering 10,000,000,000 sheets a year, of which the Japanese themselves consume an average of 96 sheets per person a year.

A Wealth of Nutrition

Throughout their long history of use, sea vegetables have always been valued for their health-giving properties. A recent study in Japan has shown that people live longer and stay healthier in the areas where sea vegetables are eaten abundantly. Common causes of death, such as cerebral haemorrhage and high blood-pressure are notably rare in these areas. The famous women pearl divers of Japan and Korea, who dive to considerable depths virtually naked throughout the year, until well past their seventieth birthdays, are careful to consume wakame, hijiki and nori each day. It is well known amongst Japanese people that regular consumption of hijiki and arame will ensure a clear complexion, soft pliant skin and thick shiny hair.

The sea is the origin of life. Millions of years of erosion of the land have enriched the sea with a wealth of all the minerals necessary for life. Sea vegetables contain between ten and twenty times the minerals of land vegetables supplying both those we need in quantity, such as calcium, iron, potassium, iodine and magnesium, and the lesser so-called 'trace' minerals for which our requirements may be minimal but without which certain essential body functions cannot perform. Iodine is difficult to obtain from any other source than the sea, and sea vegetables contain sufficient amounts to prevent goitre, an enlargement of the thyroid gland. The traditional 'goitre belt' in Britain ran from Somerset to Yorkshire, in inland areas where the people ate almost no sea vegetables.

Sea plants, in spite of their high absorption of minerals from the sea, do not generally absorb pollutants as fish do. Where the level of pollution is high, they fail to grow. The considerably reduced nori crops in some of Japan's coastal waters are evidence of this. In fact one of the nutritional characteristics of sea vegetables is their ability to actually remove radioactive and toxic metal pollutants from the body. Sea vegetables contain quantities of alginic acid, the sticky substance that holds their cells together enabling them to live in a constantly moving water environment. Recent scientific studies at McGill University in Montreal have shown that this alginic acid can bind with the toxins in our body and allow their natural elimination.

Sea vegetables are valuable foods for all vegetarians and vegans and of great benefit generally in industrialized countries where today overeating is a threat. Their abundance of minerals has an alkalizing effect on the blood and can purify the system by eliminating the acidic effects of a modern diet. They can contain up to 25 per cent more protein than milk, yet are virtually free of calories as they are low in fat and their carbohydrate is not fully absorbed. They contain many vitamins, often to comparable levels of the richest land vegetables. Vitamins contained are A, B, C, D_3, E, K and small amounts of the elusive B_{12} which rarely occurs in foods of vegetable origin. Sea vegetables can also help dissolve fat and mucous deposits that build up in the body from an overconsumption of meat, dairy products and rich foods. From a nutritional and health aspect it seems surprising that these traditional foods have not been rediscovered before.

An Abundance of Varieties

Sea plants are amongst the most ancient forms of life on earth. Throughout the long course of evolution there has been relatively little change in their ocean environment and they have retained their simple nature. Unlike land plants, their form is largely undifferentiated, showing a minimum of tissue types within each plant. Although the leaf (frond), stem (stipe), and root (holdfast) are different in shape, their tissue composition is the same. The holdfast does not extract nourishment and acts only as an anchor for the plant. Nourishment is taken through the entire plant surface directly from sea water and converted by the plant into organic compounds. Reproduction is accomplished through simple, primitive sporing. This suggests that sea plants are little advanced from being colonies of individual cells linked up for mutual benefit, hardly having changed through the long course of evolution.

In spite of their simple primitive nature, sea plants exhibit a wide range of forms. The largest, the giant Pacific kelps, have stipes several feet in diameter with fronds that stretch for hundreds of feet, which by sheer size dwarf the largest giant redwood trees. The smallest are still a collection of simple cell colonies formed together into a dense sponge-like growth. In between are a wealth of shapes, textures and forms.

All sea plants contain chlorophyll and photosynthesize according to the quantity and quality of light available. The greater the depth of the sea, the less light penetrates from the sun. The quality of this light changes as well. Deeper than thirty feet all the long wavelengths (red light) have been absorbed by the water leaving only the short wavelengths (green and blue light). This accounts for the colour of the sea. Classification of sea vegetables is by colour into green algae, brown algae and red algae. Generally green algae grow in the shallowest waters, red in the deepest and brown in between. This relationship between colour and depth is general and there are exceptions.

Sea plants, unlike their cousins on the land, grow more abundantly in colder waters and during the colder seasons. Tropical varieties are usually small, isolated, grass-like plants. In comparison, the colder seas can produce luxuriant forests of growth containing numerous varieties. Harvesting from these colder waters will often take place during the late winter or early spring, to take advantage of this abundant growth. Again, unlike land plants, almost no varieties (with the occasional tropical exception) are poisonous, and all parts of the plant are edible. The only restricting factor for use may be toughness or lack of palatability.

Similar sea vegetables from different parts of the world tend to have different qualities. Kombu, for example, from North America or Europe is usually firmer in texture and stronger flavoured than kombu from Japan, which is softer textured and sweeter to taste. This is because the ocean waters are different. The North Atlantic is more turbulent creating a tougher, richer flavoured plant and more mineralized (notably in lodine). Neither kombu is necessarily better. They are just different! Atlantic kombu may be appealing for its rich nutritional value, Japanese kombu for its delicate flavour.

Available in our shops today are a dozen or so widely different sea vegetables. They vary immensely in taste, texture and colour. There is the spicy, mineral taste of purple-red dulse, the gentle green lushness of nori and wakame, and the subtle sweetness of kombu. There is the firm, neutral-tasting gel of agar-agar and the mineral tasting gel of carragheen. There are the clean, savoury tasting threads of arame and the strongly flavoured, black strings of hijiki. Combined with other ingredients and cooked with care, sea vegetables can extend the horizons of cooking natural foods into appealing new dimensions of discovery.

A Traditional Food for the Future

The sea is one of our greatest untapped resources of food. Traditional societies were aware of this, but our realization is minimal. With increasing concern today with overpopulation and food shortages arising from an overworked and undernourished land, it is reassuring to know of the bountiful harvest lying hidden around our coastlines. In addition to this self-replenishing natural supply the potential for developing cultivation is immense. The Japanese, over the last few centuries, in order to support a growing population from a small area of farmland, have extended their farming beyond the shoreline and into the sea. They have opened our eyes to the amazing potential of off-shore farming that, if practised on a larger scale throughout the world, could in the long-term be a saviour for mankind.

Cooking with Sea Vegetables

Storage

Sea vegetables are usually available in dried form, which makes them ideal for long-term storage. To keep them in peak condition always transfer into an air-tight jar after opening the package. Nori, especially, needs to be kept very dry to preserve its flavour, so do not leave open packets lying around (very high-grade nori in Japan is always sold in sealed tins). Reputable suppliers will carefully reduce the moisture content of their sea vegetables to the optimum level before packing and you should have no problems. If they do become damp, simply dry briefly in a low oven. Occasionally white spots may form on the surface of sea vegetables during storage. These are usually crystals of salt that have been brought to the surface by a change in temperature. They can be simply wiped off before use. Because of their relative light weight and ability to keep well, sea vegetables are ideal travelling foods. We always take some packages of ready to eat or quick to prepare varieties with us when we are going on trips as a balance to the more extreme foods we may encounter. If you harvest your own sea vegetables or are fortunate enough to obtain fresh supplies (they always taste better), wash them in fresh water and store in a cool place or refrigerator. They will keep as long as fresh green land vegetables. Alternatively, dry them after washing by hanging in the sun or in a warm dry place.

Preparation

Because of their dry nature, sea vegetables expand considerably on soaking and are very economical to use. Different varieties expand to different degrees, hijiki for instance expands a lot more than arame. Experience will soon indicate the correct amount to use. It is common in the beginning to use too much. First wipe with a damp cloth to remove any surface salt, then wash quickly under the tap to remove any sand or shell particles. Soak with enough water to allow for expansion. The time of soaking will vary for different sea vegetables (see recipes for details). Retain the soaking water for use in the recipe if possible, carefully pouring it from the bowl and discarding the last part as it may contain fine sand particles. (If the soaking water is too salty, combine with fresh water.) If you are cutting when dry, scissors often work better than a knife, and they are always the easiest way to cut sheets of nori. Soaked sea vegetables are best cut with a good sharp knife on a wooden board. A Japanese vegetable cutting knife will give good results.

Cooking

Cooking is the art of mastering the ways of changing quality and energy in food. The technique lies in the controlled use of the key elements — fire, water, salt, pressure and time. The quality of the fire is important and the direct live flame of gas is preferable to the indirect energy of electricity. It is also easier to control. Aluminium pans, although cheap, are not ideal for cooking as the metal is soft and easily eroded by the acids in food, causing contamination of flavours. The best pans are stainless steel or enamel for lighter or quicker cooking, and cast iron, enamelled cast iron or earthenware for slower or longer cooking. Preferably use wooden utensils in cooking. Unlike metal, their neutral quality will harmonize, rather than conflict with, the flavour of the food. A suribachi (Japanese serrated mortar and pestle), or a hand food mill, again, is more harmonious to the food than an electric blender when you wish to purée.

Some sea vegetables are tender enough to eat raw after a brief soaking. Others need a light cooking, like boiling or steaming, whilst some require stronger cooking, like sautéing or simmering. Lighter cooking will create a dominant dispersing energy in the food more suitable to spring and summer dishes. Stronger cooking will create a dominant gathering energy more suitable to autumn and winter dishes. In our recipes we show a variety of cooking styles used according to the quality of the sea vegetable and the type of dish we wish to create. The recipes are examples and we encourage you to experiment with your own creations. Cooking with sea vegetables can be as varied and exciting as cooking with land vegetables.

Menu Planning

Because sea vegetables are very concentrated and highly nutritious, there is a temptation to take advantage of their benefits, serving large helpings occasionally, then forgetting about them for a while. Sea vegetables should ideally be eaten in small amounts but regularly. The key to their use lies in careful menu planning, attempting with each meal to create a harmonious balance of vegetable dishes centred around whole cereal grains. This traditional balance has served most societies well for centuries, only being surpassed in recent history by the tendency to allow animal foods to dominate the meal. As well as creating a balanced diet nutritionally, it is important also to create a harmonious balance with a stimulating variety of tastes, textures and colours. Here the incorporation of sea vegetables can add a new dimension, with a wealth of new sensory pleasures. Our recipes use sea vegetables in the traditional way as a small but vital ingredient in everyday cooking that hopefully will nourish in the fullest sense, being both a joy to behold and a joy to eat.

Choosing other Ingredients

In our recipes you may encounter some new ingredients. They are all traditional whole foods that have originated where vegetarian cuisine has been practised for many centuries. Most of these foods are now widely available and many are now being manufactured on a local basis. For all ingredients we recommend using a high quality source. Not only will the food be more nutritious but the taste superior to that of a lower quality source. It can be false economy to buy by price alone. By eliminating the more 'extreme' foods from our diet: meat, cheese, butter, eggs, coffee, tropical fruits, sugar, etc., foods that place undue stress on our system by their excessively expanding, contracting or fatty nature — and using some of the cost savings to buy higher quality vegetarian ingredients, we receive a balanced diet that is more nourishing and less taxing on our body. It can also be less taxing on the pocket as you can end up paying far less than the national average on your weekly food bill. Before the days of consumer affluence simple folk with their daily fare of whole cereal grains and vegetables usually maintained a sound robust health. Incidences of cancer, heart conditions and other degenerative diseases directly correlate to the extent that 'extreme' foods are eaten today by our society.

Cereal Grains

Preferably use whole cereal grains, cooked in their whole form, rather than as flakes or flour. Whole grains still contain their full energy value and are most nourishing and digestible when chewed well. Select from a variety of the temperate cereal grains — rice, barley, oats, wheat, rye, millet, buckwheat and maize. Brown rice is the most popular of all cereal grains and for temperate climates, short and medium grain varieties are more suitable. Long grain, patna-style rice is a tropical grain and generally too light for temperate climates. Sweet brown rice (glutinous rice) has a delightfully sweet and sticky quality and is a very warming and strengthening food. It is available from all good natural food stores. *Soba* and *udon* are two traditional Japanese noodles that are a delight to use. *Soba* is made from buckwheat and wheat and *udon* from wholewheat. They are made with softer wheat than Italian style wholewheat pasta and we find them lighter and more digestible.

Dried Beans and Bean Products

The protein of beans is a nutritional complement to that of whole grains. Together they can provide a complete balance of all the essential amino acids without resort to animal foods. For regular use choose the smaller or more compact varieties, like aduki beans, chickpeas, and lentils. Thorough cooking is always essential with beans to make them fully digestible and cooking with kombu will make them softer and more nutritious. Soya beans especially, although they are extremely rich in protein and natural fats, can be indigestible unless thoroughly cooked. For this reason, throughout their long history of use in the Far East, they have invariably been processed or fermented before use to allow for ready assimilation of their nutrients. Several of these products are now becoming popular in the West and we use them freely in our recipes. Here is a brief summary of the most common ones.

Soya Sauce — *Shoyu* and *tamari* are Japanese names for natural soya sauce. Choose a reputable brand that contains only whole ingredients and has been naturally aged over two summers in wooden kegs at ambient temperature. A natural soya sauce will be rich and mellow with none of the harshness found in cheaper brands that can be little more than chemical cocktails. Read labels carefully — a good natural sauce will always indicate the production method on the label. *Shoyu* is fermented from soya beans, wheat and sea salt whilst *tamari* contains just soya and sea salt. *Shoyu* has a richer flavour, is cheaper, and most recommended for everyday seasoning. *Tamari* is thicker, more mellow and more expensive, and has traditionally been used for special dip sauces. Natural soya sauce is an invaluable seasoning and contains a wealth of easily digestible nutrients.

Miso — This close relative of soya sauce is a rich brown purée of soya beans fermented with sea salt and usually a cereal grain. Look for a brand that has been made to the same high standards indicated for natural soya sauce. Barley, *mugi miso*, is most suitable for everyday use. Brown rice, *genmai miso*, is a lighter variety popular in summer cooking. Miso is a perfect base for soups and sauces and, along with natural soya sauce, is an important food for vegetarians, containing a complete and readily assimilable protein along with a good balance of carbohydrates, fats, minerals and vitamins. Both contain small quantities of vitamin B_{12} that is naturally produced during fermentation.

Tofu — is an ancient food from the Far East that is made from soya beans and has a light cheese-like quality. It is now becoming very popular in the West being increasingly made and distributed on a local scale. Its mild flavour lends it to a variety of combinations with other foods.

Tempeh — is another traditional vegetarian soya bean fermentation, originating in Indonesia, and also becoming well known in the West. Its firm texture and pleasing flavour lend it to a variety of uses. Tempeh is the richest vegetarian source of naturally occurring vitamin B_{12}.

Natto — The taste of these sticky fermented soya beans is either loved or hated. It is somewhat like a very ripe cheese. Natto is usually served in small amounts with grated raw carrot, or daikon, or mustard and seasoned with shoyu. It is an attractive condiment with brown rice. Natto is available in good wholefood and Japanese stores.

Seitan — Although not a bean product but the gluten of wheat, seitan, is another traditional vegetarian food that is becoming increasingly popular in the West. It is available in good wholefood stores and can also be easily made at home. It is prepared from hard wheat flour that is well kneaded and washed to remove the starch, then cooked in water seasoned with shoyu, ginger and kombu.

With the increase in availability of these high quality natural vegetarian proteins it is well worth discovering and using them, rather than relying on commercial textured soya proteins and pâtés that are mass produced and invariably contain added colouring and flavouring.

Vegetables and Fruits

Buy organically grown vegetables and fruits when available. They are often a little more expensive, but their flavour, deriving from their more balanced nutrition, is usually better. Not only are you avoiding chemicals, but you are encouraging a balanced agriculture that will benefit our society for generations to come. Try to use only local and seasonal vegetables and fruits. If they have grown in the same environment as us they will help us adapt to the local climate and season. Tropical fruit may make us feel at home in the tropics but not in a cold northern winter!

Daikon — is a long white radish that is perfect for cooking. In Britain it is becoming increasingly easy to obtain and is usually sold under the name *mooli*. It can generally be found in good vegetable markets.

Burdock — is one of the most strengthening of all root vegetables. It grows deep into the soil and has a pleasantly bitter taste. Although it can be bought in some wholefood stores, it can always be found growing wild on waste land both in cities and in the country.

Shiitake mushrooms — are a dried variety from Japan prized for their delicate flavour. Before cooking, soak for 10-15 minutes until soft, discarding the harder parts of the stem.

Condiments and Seasonings

Salt — A natural additive-free sea salt is preferable to commercial refined salt. It contains the full balance of trace elements and has a more mellow and less burning taste.

Oil — Choose an unrefined vegetable oil. Oil is a food and not just a lubricant! You can recognize an unrefined oil by its rich natural colour and full flavour indicating that its nutritional value has not been dissolved, bleached and deodorized away by the chemicals used in commercial oil production. Preferably use unrefined sesame oil, or if you require a stronger flavour, toasted sesame oil.

Umeboshi — These salt pickled plums from Japan have a uniquely tart and tangy taste that enhances a variety of savoury dishes. They are prized for their highly alkaline properties and need only be used in small amounts. They are also available in purée form.

Kuzu — A natural wild mountain root starch from Japan that is an ideal thickening agent and is used like arrowroot for clear sauces and glazes. It is rich in minerals and highly digestible and is often used as a medicinal food for the digestive system.

Tahini — This purée of creamed sesame seeds is a traditional Mediterranean food. Choose a natural brand without added oil. *Sesame spread*, otherwise known as *sesame butter*, is a more coarsely ground and salted alternative, that is also available in wholefood stores.

Vinegar — *Brown rice vinegar* is an ideal vinegar being pleasantly mild, mellow tasting, and a perfect complement to grain and vegetable dishes. A good quality *apple cider vinegar* is an alternative, but being sharper and stronger, will be needed in smaller amounts. *Ume-su*, red plum seasoning, is the natural juice from umeboshi that can also be used like vinegar as a dressing for vegetables and salads.

Ginger — The juice squeezed from freshly grated roots is always preferable to powdered ginger. If not available, ensure your ginger powder is as fresh as possible.

Wasabi — is a green coloured root of a Japanese plant with a hot taste similar to mustard or horseradish. It adds a wonderful perk to dishes and can sometimes be preferable to mustard. It is available in powder form in good wholefood and Japanese stores. Substitute a natural mustard or natural horseradish if unavailable.

On Using Natural Sweeteners

What is sold as sugar is basically sucrose, an extremely sweet simple sugar that can upset the metabolism by depleting the body's mineral supply and weakening the quality of the blood. It has a reputation as a vicious destroyer of teeth and it can only be viewed as a non-nutritive short term energy booster. Whether it is brown or white, raw or highly processed, makes very little difference to its effect on the body. In the interests of health, and to prevent a dose of the notorious 'sugar blues', it is best avoided in any form.

With so-called natural sweeteners, it is also best to proceed with caution. Fruits derive their sweetness from the abundant presence of the simple sugars fructose and sucrose, and although they may be natural and unprocessed, in tropical varieties or in a concentrated form, they too can have a powerful and damaging effect on the body.

Honey, although it is naturally produced from nectar (plant sucrose) by the digestive system of bees, contains about 80 per cent simple sugars that again, in quantity, can cause a severe jolt to the system. Honey, also, is strongly flavoured and tends to overpower the natural taste of food it is combined with. Maple syrup, as well, although entirely of vegetable origin (the simply cooked-down sap of maple trees), is another powerhouse of sucrose, containing about 65 per cent by weight.

The best way to obtain sweetness is to thoroughly chew cooked whole grains and vegetables. The longer they are chewed the sweeter they taste as their complex sugars break down with the saliva into simpler sugars. The body then absorbs them naturally and slowly without unbalancing the system. When added sweetness is desired in a dish, try using a naturally processed cereal sweetener like barley malt (malt extract), rice syrup, amazake, maltose, or mirin (a sweet cooking liquid made from rice and primarily used for sweetening savoury dishes). Through enzymatic or yeast action during processing the complex starches have been reduced to maltose and glucose, the simple sugars that have the least damaging effect on the teeth and the body. The taste of cereal sweeteners is also relatively mild and harmonizes readily with other grain and vegetable quality foods.

Vegetable Cutting

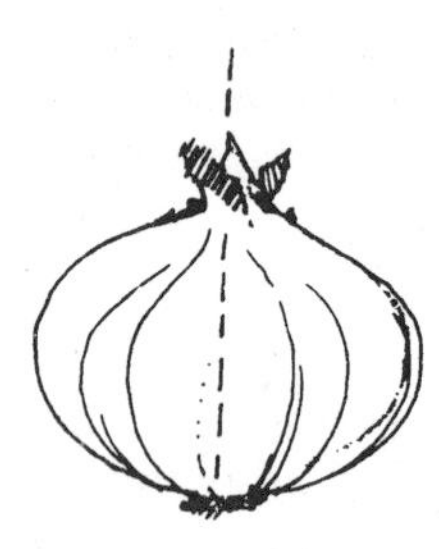

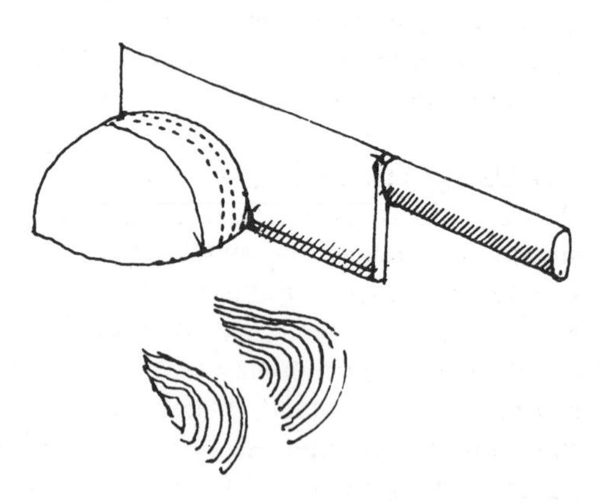

Onions Cut into Half Moons

1. Peel the outer dry skin off the onion and trim off the top and root.

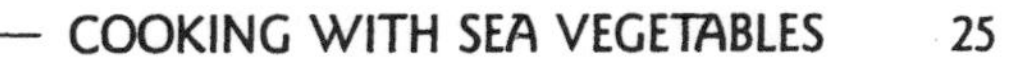

2. Make one vertical cut down through the onion.
3. Lay each half down and make vertical cuts to give thin slices.

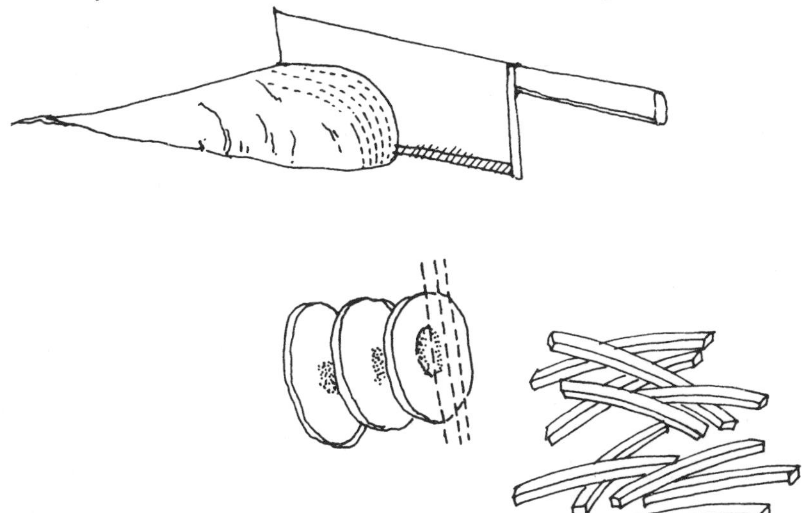

Matchsticks

1. Wash the vegetable thoroughly to remove any remaining dirt.
2. By cutting vertically on the diagonal make thin slices.
3. Lay these down and cut into thin matchsticks.

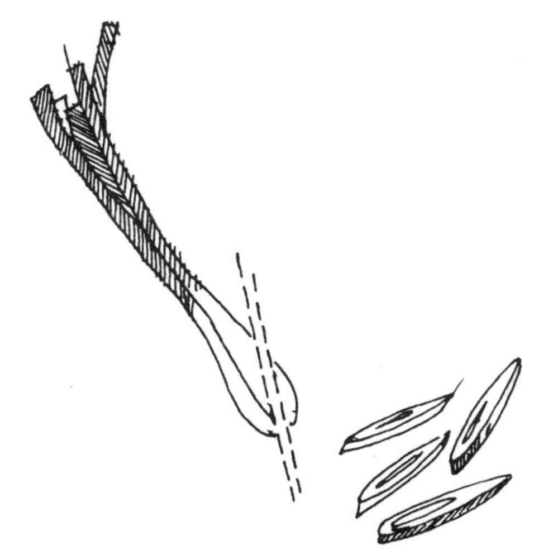

Cutting on the Diagonal

1. Wash the vegetable thoroughly and trim off any dead parts.
2. By cutting vertically on the diagonal make thin slices.

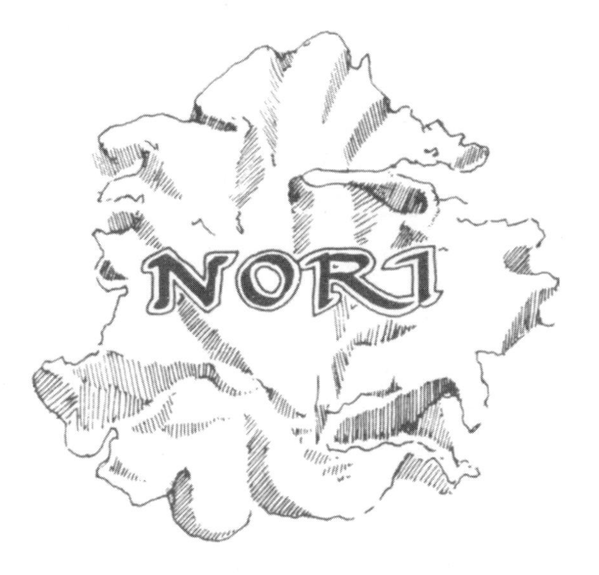

Nori, or laver as it is commonly known in the West, is the most popular of all sea vegetables, being quick and easy to prepare and lending itself to a wide variety of uses. It is also probably the most palatable for newcomers, having a mild flavour. This mildness derives from its preferred habitat, close to the shore line in sheltered inlets, where fresh water from rivers dilutes the saltiness of the sea. Nori is one of the richest sea vegetable sources of protein and also contains large amounts of vitamins C and B_1, and is especially rich in vitamin A, containing as much as some carrots. Because it can decrease cholesterol in the body by helping to break down and eliminate fat deposits, nori is especially beneficial to people with a background of heavy dairy food eating. It is also an aid to digestion and is often served in combination with fried foods.

Nori is usually sold dried in sheet form, with ten 7 inch (18cm) square sheets folded per package. Sheet nori comes almost entirely from Japan where it is the product of a large industry employing over 300,000 people (one quarter of the total number of people employed in agriculture in Britain). Unlike other sea vegetables production is entirely from cultivated plants. In early autumn bamboo poles are set in a grid pattern into the muddy bottoms of bays around the coast. Meanwhile on the shore, spores are being cultivated in special tanks which are then transferred onto rope nets that are hung between the poles in the water. Optimum growth is achieved by positioning the nets at such a height so they remain above the water level during low tide, to gain maximum sunlight, yet receive a regular washing below the water level during high tide. During the winter, after a few months of growth, the mature plants are harvested either by hand picking or by a suction pump.

The fresh harvested nori is then washed, finely chopped into a thick soupy mix, and ladled in measured amounts into a frame on bamboo mats. The excess liquid drains away and the nori-coated mats are then simply dried, either in the traditional way outside in the sun, or more commonly nowadays, indoors in large ovens. The thin sheets of nori which result are then peeled off the mats, folded and packaged, each sheet having embossed on its surface the noticeable impression of the drying mat.

Sheet nori can vary considerably both in price and quality with a higher price generally reflecting a higher quality, although for the very expensive grades (usually sold in tins in Japanese food shops) your money is not buying an increase in nutrition, merely a subtle improvement in the delicacy of the flavour. A good grade nori will be somewhat brittle and shiny and when held up to the light should have an overall green translucency with an even texture. Beware of cheap grades, which can be purple, limp and uneven. They may also be artificially dyed green and chemically lacquered. Sheet nori is also available ready-toasted in flat sheets, known as *sushi nori,* or toasted and shredded into fine strips for garnishing, known as *kizami nori.* To preserve the delicate flavour and prevent moisture absorption, always keep nori in a dry sealed container. Sheet nori is most commonly toasted briefly before use by waving over a flame until the colour changes to a bright green. It can then be cut into strips for using as a garnish or as a wrapper for rice balls and sushi rolls. These nori-covered foods are the oriental equivalent of our western sandwich.

Many types of nori grow wild in different parts of the world. At the time of writing, though, nori is not cultivated, nor is it prepared into sheets outside the Far East. Wild nori may vary in colour from bright green, through olive green, to brown, purple or black according to its age and degree of exposure to light. Around the British Isles it is known as *laver* in Wales, *sloke* in Ireland, *slake* in Scotland, and *black butter* in Devon. Traditionally it has been cooked down into a thick purée (*laverbread* in Wales) and served as a condiment, often with oatmeal. Our nori condiment recipe is in this tradition. Wild nori contains more minerals, is stronger tasting, and is slightly tougher than cultivated nori. Nori condiment prepared from sheet nori will have a lighter, more delicate flavour.

Green Nori Flakes *(ao-nori)* are from a different variety of sea vegetable whose bright green flakes are ready-to-eat and make a tasty herb-like condiment for garnishing a variety of dishes.

Purple Leaf Nori *(fu-nori)* is a sea vegetable that is very soft and delicate. It requires almost no cooking and is a delight in soups, salads and vinegared dishes. Coarser varieties of *fu-nori* were traditionally used in Japan as a natural hair shampoo.

Sea Lettuce is a light green leafy vegetable that has long been used in Britain by simply boiling and serving as a vegetable. It also makes a wonderfully rich dry condiment when toasted and crushed into fine flakes.

Nori Soup with Sheet Nori

Serves 4-5

Imperial (Metric)	American
Few drops of sesame oil	Few drops of sesame oil
6 oz (170g) onions, cut into half moons	1 cup onions, cut into half moons
Few drops of shoyu	Few drops of shoyu
3 oz (85g) fresh mushrooms, finely sliced	1 cup fresh mushrooms, finely sliced
2 pints (1.1 litres) water	5 cups water
2 sheets of nori	2 sheets of nori
5 tablespoons shoyu	5 tablespoons shoyu
Spring onions, chopped to garnish	Scallions, chopped to garnish

1. Brush a deep pot with a small amount of sesame oil and heat. Add the onions and sauté for 3 minutes on a medium heat, adding a few drops of shoyu while sautéing. Add the mushrooms and sauté for a further 2-3 minutes.
2. Add the water and bring to the boil.
3. Break the nori sheets into small pieces and add to the soup. Simmer for 5 minutes.
4. Add the shoyu and simmer for 1-2 minutes. Serve garnished with the chopped spring onions (scallions).

Note: This is a very quick to prepare and delicious soup.

Nori Wrapped Rice Balls

Makes 2 rice balls

Imperial (Metric)	American
1 sheet of nori	1 sheet of nori
9 oz (255g) cooked brown rice	1½ cups cooked brown rice
1 umeboshi plum	1 umeboshi plum

1. Toast the sheet of nori (shiny side up) by holding it horizontally 10 inches (25cm) above a gas flame and rotating it for a few seconds until its colour changes to bright green. Fold the sheet in half and then half again so it breaks into four equal sized pieces.
2. Wet your hands to prevent the rice sticking to them, then take half the amount of rice and by cupping your hands together and pressing form the rice into a firm ball.
3. Press a hole into the middle with your thumb and place a small piece of the umeboshi plum inside so it is right in the centre of the ball. Pack the ball closed again and by cupping action slightly flatten the top and bottom of the ball. Repeat to make the second rice ball.
4. With thoroughly dry hands, place one square of nori on the top and one square on the bottom of each rice ball. Position centrally and have the corners of the top square over the side of the bottom square, so when wrapped around all the corners dovetail between each other (see Figure 5).
5. Press the nori with cupped hands firmly onto the rice, cutting off overlapping nori and using to fill any gaps. Continue pressing the nori firmly for about 1 minute until well stuck on to the rice.

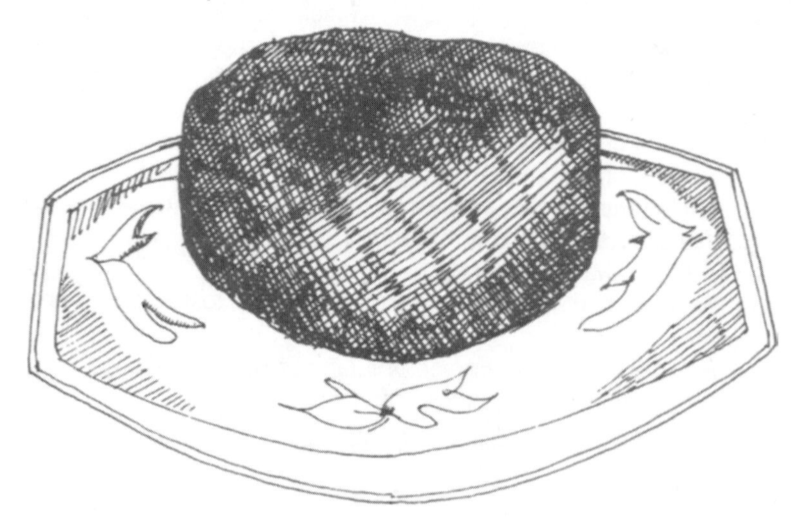

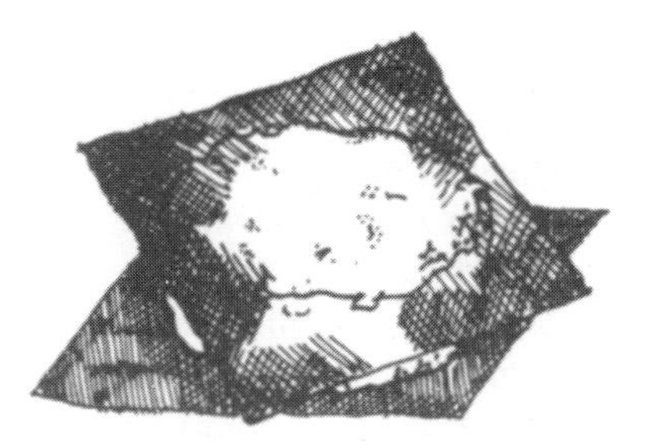

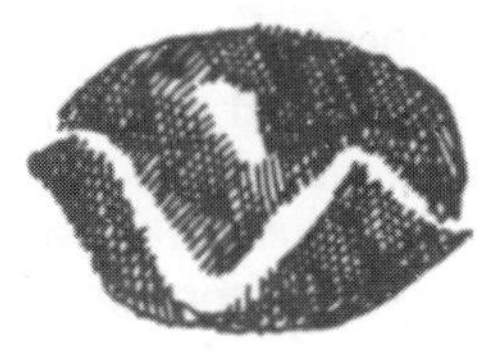

Variation:

Nori Rice Triangles

Ingredients as for Nori Wrapped Rice Balls (page 30).

1. Shape the rice as for rice balls, fill with pieces of umeboshi and close up. Form with the hands into triangles rather than rounds but again with a flattened top and bottom.
2. Toast the nori sheet as for rice balls and cut into 1 inch (2.5cm) strips. With dry hands place a strip around the sides of the triangles leaving the flattened top and bottom open. Press on firmly, sticking the overlapping ends of the nori strip together with a drop of water if necessary.

Note: To make good rice balls use rice that is slightly moist and holds together well. Rice that is either too dry or too wet will not produce good results. When forming the rice balls it is necessary to have wet hands but when covering with nori your hands need to be thoroughly dry. If the nori becomes too moist the balls will spoil easily. The umeboshi inside each rice ball (salty pickles can also be used) as well as being a tasty seasoning also acts as a natural preservative. Well-made rice balls can keep for several days and are very useful for travelling and for packed lunches and picnics. In Japan they are a national dish and the equivalent of our sandwich. They are a well balanced and wholesome food and alone can make a very satisfying lunch. To pack rice balls for travelling wrap them in a sushi mat or a paper bag where they can breathe without drying out excessively. Cling film or polythene can cause them to sweat and spoil easily.

Sushi Nori Rolls (Nori Maki) I

Makes 6-8 pieces

Imperial (Metric)	American
1 sheet of nori	1 sheet of nori
9 oz (255g) cooked brown rice, allowed to cool slightly	1½ cups cooked brown rice, allowed to cool slightly
1 tablespoon sesame spread	1 tablespoon sesame butter
½ tablespoon umeboshi paste	½ tablespoon umeboshi paste
Strips of carrot, ¼-½ inch (5-10mm) thick and wide, boiled for 1 minute with a pinch of sea salt	Strips of carrot, ¼-½ inch thick and wide, boiled for 1 minute with a pinch of sea salt

1. Toast the sheet of nori by holding it horizontally 10 inches (25cm) above a gas flame and rotating it for a few seconds until the colour changes to bright green.
2. Place the toasted sheet of nori on a bamboo sushi mat with the stripping of the mat running from left to right. Spread the cooked brown rice evenly on the nori but leaving a clear ½ inch (1cm) at the top and bottom (see Figure 6).

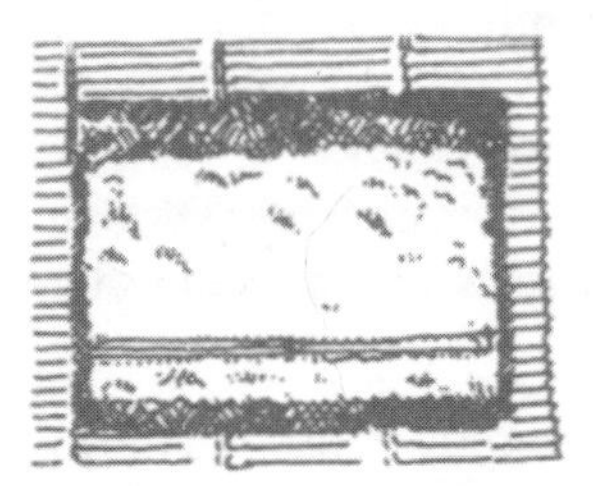

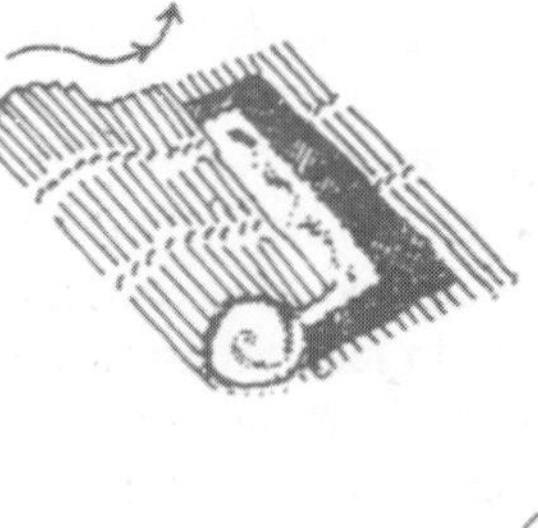

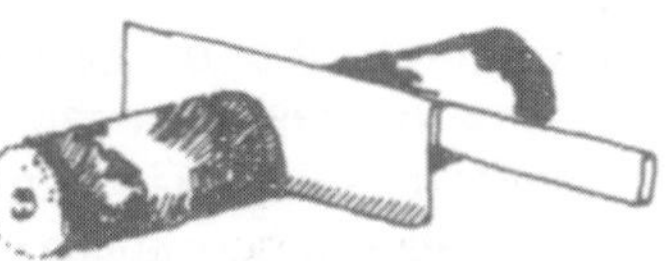

3. Make an indentation in the rice with a chopstick running from left to right across the centre of the rice. Fill this with the sesame spread (sesame butter) and umeboshi paste and then place the carrot strips along it.
4. From the bottom, start rolling up the sushi mat around the ingredients, pressing it firmly onto the nori. Whilst rolling, slowly pull the leading edge of the mat back so it does not roll into the sushi.
5. Continue rolling until the uncovered end of the nori is reached, then wet this edge and complete rolling to seal the sushi. A final gentle squeeze of the mat around the sushi will ensure a tight roll.
6. To prevent the sushi drying out, cut just before serving. With a sharp knife slice the roll across in half and then each half into 3 or 4 rounds.

Notes to Sushi Making: There is a knack to making good sushi and this can easily be learnt with practice. The key is the quality of the cooked rice. This should be slightly sticky and freshly cooked. It should be fairly cool but still containing some warmth. Take time to spread the rice evenly over the nori and to position the filling ingredients carefully. When rolling go slowly, ensuring that the filling does not spill out of the ends. If the ends do come out a little ragged, they can be trimmed off before cutting.

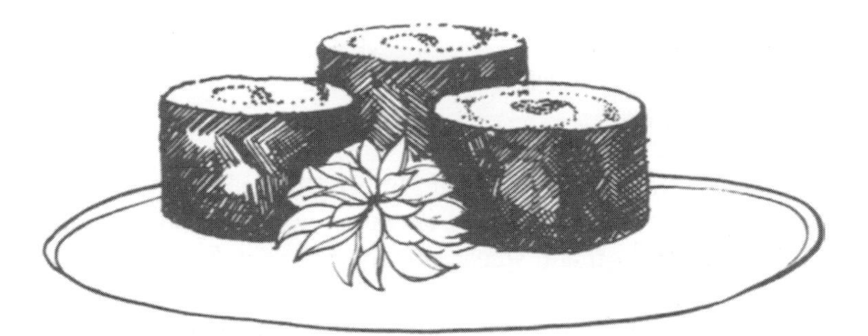

Sushi Nori Rolls (Nori Maki) II

Makes 6-8 pieces

Imperial (Metric)	American
1 sheet of nori	1 sheet of nori
9 oz (225g) cooked brown rice, allowed to cool slightly	1½ cups cooked brown rice, allowed to cool slightly
1 tablespoon wasabi powder diluted with a few drops of water to make a paste	1 tablespoon wasabi powder diluted with a few drops of water to make a paste
1 seven-inch (18cm) long strip cucumber, ¼-½ inch (5-10mm) thick and wide	1 seven-inch long strip cucumber, ¼-½ inch thick and wide

1. Prepare the sushi as Recipe 1, substituting the wasabi paste for sesame spread.

Note: Natural mustard or horseradish can be used instead of wasabi.

Sushi Nori Rolls (Nori Maki) III

Makes 6-8 pieces

Imperial (Metric)	American
1½ oz (45g) seitan wheat gluten	¼ cup seitan wheat meat
Sesame.oil, for deep frying	Sesame oil, for deep frying
1 sheet of nori	1 sheet of nori
9 oz (255g) cooked brown rice, allowed to cool slightly	1½ cups cooked brown rice, allowed to cool slightly
1 tablespoon natural mustard	1 tablespoon natural mustard
¼ teaspoon shoyu	¼ teaspoon shoyu

1. Deep fry the seitan in the oil at 350°F/180°C for 2-3 minutes. Drain on a paper towel to remove excess oil. Cut into fine strips.
2. Prepare the nori and spread out the rice as in Sushi Nori Rolls I (page 32).
3. Mix the mustard and shoyu together and spread over the rice.
4. Place the strips of seitan in the indentation across the rice.
5. Complete rolling the sushi.

Sushi Nori Rolls (Nori Maki) IV

Makes 6-8 pieces

Imperial (Metric)	American
1 sheet of nori	1 sheet of nori
9 oz (255g) cooked brown rice, allowed to cool slightly	1½ cups cooked brown rice, allowed to cool slightly
8 fl oz (230ml) water	1 cup water
½ tablespoon barley (mugi) miso	½ tablespoon barley (mugi) miso
1 tablespoon barley malt	1 tablespoon barley malt
1 seven-inch (18cm) strip daikon radish, ½ inch (10mm) wide and ¼ inch (5mm) thick	1 seven-inch strip daikon radish, ½ inch wide and ¼ inch thick

1. Prepare the sushi as in Sushi Nori Rolls I (page 32).
2. Bring the water to the boil, add the miso and barley malt, mixing well until dissolved. Add the daikon strip and cook on a medium heat for 10-15 minutes until all the water has evaporated.
3. Place the daikon strip in an indentation across the rice and roll up the sushi.

Sushi Nori Rolls (Nori Maki) V

Makes 6-8 pieces

Imperial (Metric)	American
1 sheet of nori	1 sheet of nori
9 oz (255g) cooked brown rice, allowed to cool slightly	1½ cups cooked brown rice, allowed to cool slightly
Pickles (any kind) cut into ¼ inch by ¼ inch strips	Pickles (any kind) cut into ¾ inch by ¼ inch strips.

1. Follow the method for Sushi Nori Rolls I, substituting the pickles for the carrots.

The varieties of sushi are endless and these recipes are just a few examples. Experiment with your own favourite combinations, remembering to keep the tastes simple and clear. Presentation is part of the enjoyment of these foods and it is worth spending some time making attractive displays. Sushi make a perfect party food and can be used for snacks, packed lunches and for travelling, as well as being served as part of a daily meal.

Nori Rolls with Soba and Sauerkraut (Soba Maki)

Makes 6-8 pieces

Imperial (Metric)	American
1 sheet of nori	1 sheet of nori
½ packet soba (buckwheat spaghetti)	½ package soba (buckwheat noodles)
Sesame oil, a few drops	Sesame oil, a few drops
2 oz (55g) sauerkraut	½ cup sauerkraut
Few drops shoyu	Few drops shoyu
1 spring onion, boiled for ½ minute with a pinch of sea salt	1 scallion, boiled for ½ minute with a pinch of sea salt

1. Toast the sheet of nori by holding it horizontally 10 inches (25cm) above a gas flame and rotating it for 3-5 seconds until its colour changes to a bright green.
2. Cook the soba in boiling water without salt. They are cooked when the inside and outside are the same colour. Rinse under cold water to cool. Drain and dry lightly by pressing with a cloth.
3. Place the soba carefully on the toasted nori with all the strands running from left to right. Leave a gap at the top and bottom as with rice sushi (see Figure 7).
4. Brush a frying pan with a small amount of sesame oil. Sauté the sauerkraut for 2-3 minutes, adding a few drops of shoyu. Allow to cool and place evenly on the soba.
5. Lay the spring onion (scallion) across the top and roll up within a sushi mat as described in the sushi recipe (page 32).
6. Serve sliced into lengths and display the ends uppermost on a flat plate.

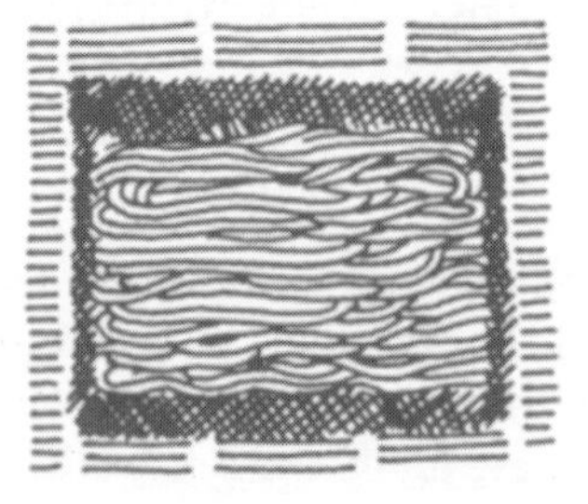

* The standard weight of a packet is 250g in the UK and Europe, and 8 oz in the USA. Either size could be used in this recipe.

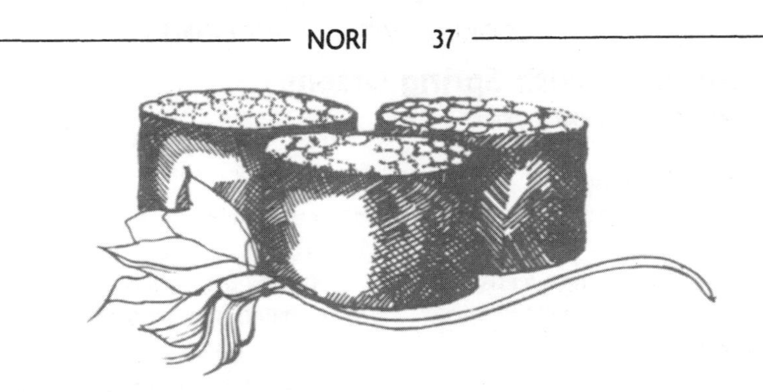

Nori Rolls with Udon and Tempeh (Udon Maki)

Makes 6-8 pieces

Imperial (Metric)	American
1 strip kombu, 3 inches long	1 strip kombu, 3 inches long
2 oz (55g) tempeh, cut into 2 strips	2 ounces tempeh, cut into 2 strips
½ tablespoon shoyu	½ tablespoon shoyu
Sesame oil for deep frying	Sesame oil for deep frying
⅓ packet udon, wholewheat spaghetti*	⅓ package udon, wholewheat noodles*
1 sheet of nori	1 sheet of nori
1 tablespoon natural mustard	1 tablespoon natural mustard

1. Place the kombu in the bottom of a heavy pot, cover with water and soak for 1 hour. Add the tempeh and shoyu, seeing that the tempeh is just half covered with water, and cook for 20 minutes on a medium heat or until the water evaporates.
2. Heat 2-3 inches of the oil in a pot to 350°F/180°C, ensuring it does not smoke.
3. Carefully drop the cooked tempeh into the hot oil. Deep fry for 1-2 minutes until the colour changes. Remove and drain on a paper towel.
4. Cook the udon in boiling water, rinse under cold water and lightly dry with a cloth.
5. Toast the sheet of nori as for Soba Maki (page 36) and lay it on a sushi mat. Cover with the udon noodles carefully ranged from left to right, leaving a gap at the top and bottom. Spread the mustard evenly over the noodles and lay the fried tempeh in a strip across the top. Roll up as described on page 33.
6. Serve sliced into lengths and display the ends uppermost on a flat plate.

Nori Rolls with Spring Greens

Makes 6-8 pieces.

Imperial (Metric)	American
1½ pints (850ml) water	3¾ cups water
Pinch sea salt	Pinch sea salt
½ lb (225g) spring greens, washed and separated into whole leaves	½ pound greens, washed and separated into whole leaves
1 sheet of nori	1 sheet of nori
Sesame seeds, roasted (optional) to garnish	Sesame seeds, roasted (optional) to garnish

1. Bring the water to the boil, add a pinch of sea salt and the greens and boil for 2-3 minutes. Remove and rinse for a few seconds under the cold tap. Drain and carefully dry with a towel to remove excess water. Spread the leaves out and cut each one in half dividing along the centre removing the stems and keeping separate.
2. Toast the sheet of nori by holding it 10 inches (25cm) above a gas flame and lay on a sushi mat. Cover with 2-3 layers of the cooked green leaves. Lay the separated stems in the centre from left to right on the top. Roll up within the sushi mat as described on page 33.
3. Cut the roll with a sharp knife into 1½ inch (4cm) lengths.
4. Stand each piece upright on a serving dish and if desired garnish each top end with a few roasted sesame seeds.

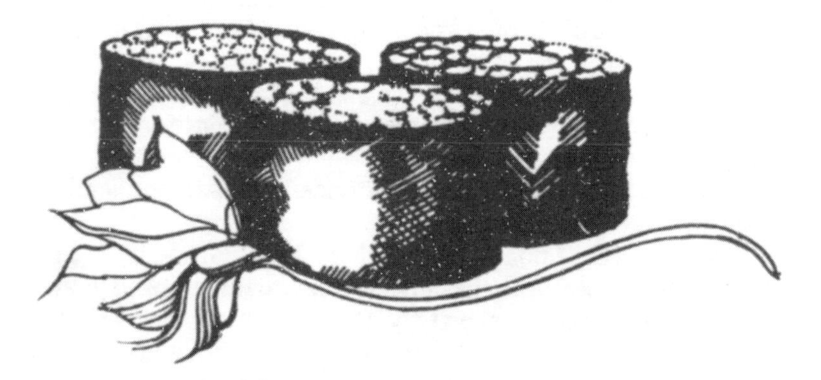

Nori Rolls with Cucumber

Makes 6-8 pieces.

Imperial (Metric)

½ cucumber, cut into long strips ¼ inch (5mm) thick and wide
¼ teaspoon sea salt
½ sheet of nori
2 oz (55g) sauerkraut
1 red radish, cut in fine matchsticks

American

½ cucumber, cut into long strips ¼ inch thick and wide
¼ teaspoon sea salt
½ sheet of nori
½ cup sauerkraut
1 red radish, cut in fine matchsticks

1. Place the cucumber strips on a plate and sprinkle with the sea salt. Leave for 1-2 hours. Dry on a towel to remove excess water.
2. Toast the half sheet of nori and lay across a sushi mat. Place the cucumber strips lengthwise across the nori. Squeeze out excess water from the sauerkraut and lay on top of the cucumber with a few of the radish matchsticks.
3. Roll up as described on page 33, cut, and serve standing upright on a flat dish.

Note: These rolls will be thinner than those in other recipes, as only half a sheet of nori is used.

Stuffed Nori Cones

Makes 8 cones

Imperial (Metric)	American
2 sheets of nori	2 sheets of nori
6 oz (170g) cooked brown rice	1 cup cooked brown rice
1 oz (30g) chopped watercress	½ cup chopped watercress
4 oz (115g) grated carrots	½ cup grated carrots
4 tablespoons roasted sesame seeds	4 tablespoons roasted sesame seeds
1 tablespoon lemon juice	1 tablespoon lemon juice
1 tablespoon natural mustard	1 tablespoon natural mustard
1 tablespoon umeboshi vinegar	1 tablespoon umeboshi vinegar
Sprigs of watercress to garnish	Sprigs of watercress to garnish

1. Toast the sheets of nori by holding shiny side up horizontally 10 inches (25cm) above a gas flame rotating until they change colour to a bright green (3-5 seconds).
2. With scissors cut each sheet into quarters. Taking one piece at a time, carefully fold into a cone shape, sticking the overlapping sides together with a drop of water.
3. Place all the remaining ingredients in a bowl and mix together.
4. Just before serving, fill each cone with the mix decorating the top of each one with a sprig of watercress.
5. Arrange neatly on a tray and serve.

Note: These cones make an attractive snack, party food or starter for a meal.

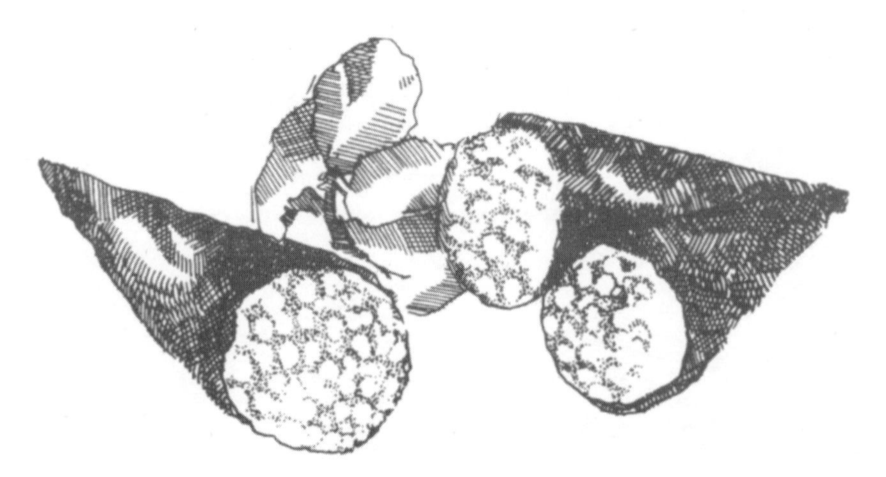

Nori Tempura

Serves 2

Imperial (Metric)	American
1 sheet of nori	1 sheet of nori
Sesame oil for deep frying	Sesame oil for deep frying
Tempura Batter:	*Tempura Batter:*
4 tablespoons wholemeal pastry flour	4 tablespoons wholewheat pastry flour
2 tablespoons maize flour	2 tablespoons cornmeal
1 tablespoon arrowroot	1 tablespoon arrowroot
Pinch of sea salt	Pinch of sea salt
Sparkling water or beer	Sparkling water or beer
Dip Sauce:	*Dip Sauce:*
1 tablespoon juice from freshly grated ginger root	1 tablespoon juice from freshly grated ginger root
½ tablespoon shoyu	½ tablespoon shoyu
5 tablespoons water	5 tablespoons water

1. Cut the nori sheet into eight 1¾ inch by 3½ inch (4.5 by 9cm) rectangles with a pair of scissors.
2. Combine all the dry ingredients for the batter then add enough sparkling water or beer to give a thick consistency. Leave to stand for at least ½ hour, ideally in a refrigerator which will produce a crispier tempura.
3. Prepare the dip sauce by combining all the ingredients.
4. Heat 2-3 inches of oil in a pan to 350°F/180°C, taking care not to let it smoke. To test the temperature, drop a small piece of batter into the oil; it should immediately sink then quickly rise to float on the surface.
5. Take one strip of nori at a time and dip it half into the batter then drop it into the oil turning it and cooking for 1-2 minutes until it turns golden brown. Drain on a paper towel.
6. Serve whilst hot, dipping each piece in the sauce before eating.

Deep Fried Tofu Wrapped in Nori

Serves 2

Imperial (Metric)

½ lb (225g) block of tofu
6 tablespoons arrowroot
1 sheet of nori, cut into 1 inch (2.5cm) wide strips
Sesame oil for deep frying
Spring onions, chopped to garnish

Sauce:

½ teaspoon shoyu
1 tablespoon juice from freshly grated ginger root
5 tablespoons water

American

½ pound block of tofu
6 tablespoons arrowroot
1 sheet of nori, cut into 1 inch wide strips
Sesame oil for deep frying
Scallions, chopped to garnish

Sauce:

½ teaspoon shoyu
1 tablespoon juice from freshly grated ginger root
5 tablespoons water

1. Place the block of tofu on a wooden cutting board and cover with a tea towel. Place a weight or plate on top to squeeze out the excess liquid from the tofu. Leave for 20 minutes, then slice into 6 rectangles. Lightly coat each piece with arrowroot and place a strip of nori around the middle of each piece, sticking the ends together with a drop of water.

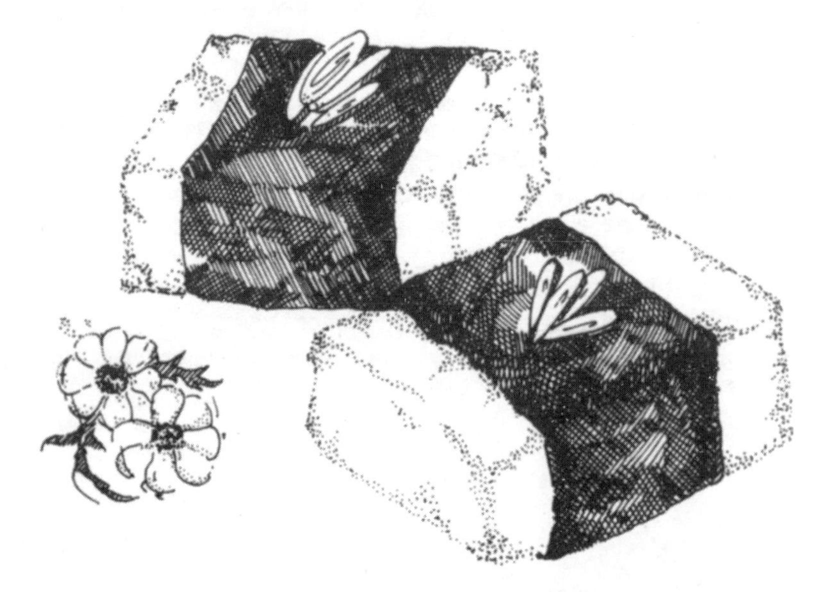

3. Heat 2-3 inches of sesame oil to 350°F/180°C and deep fry the tofu pieces until golden brown. Do not fry too many at once as this will lower the temperature of the oil. Remove from the oil and place on a paper towel to drain off the excess oil.
3. Prepare the sauce by mixing the ingredients together and then pour over the fried tofu. Garnish with the chopped spring onions (scallions). Serve hot in individual bowls with 2 or 3 pieces per person.

Tofu 'Cheese' Wrapped in Nori

Imperial (Metric)	American
½ lb (225g) block of tofu	½ pound block of tofu
Brown rice (genmai) miso	Brown rice (genmai) miso
½ sheet of nori, toasted and cut into strips	½ sheet of nori, toasted and cut into strips

1. Wrap the tofu in a tea towel and place on a wooden cutting board. Put a weight or plate on top to squeeze out the excess liquid. Leave for ½ hour.
2. Unwrap the tofu and cover all around with a ¼ inch layer of the miso. Put on a plate and store in the refrigerator for 24 hours to pickle into 'cheese'. The longer it is left the saltier it will become.
3. When pickled, remove all the miso and keep for seasoning soups. Rinse the tofu block under warm water to clean off any remaining miso. Leave to drain.
4. Cut the tofu into cubes or squares and wrap a strip of nori around each piece, sticking the overlapping ends with a drop of water if necessary.
5. Arrange attractively on a plate and serve.

Note: This dish makes an ideal party food, sandwich ingredient snack or side dish and tastes remarkably like a mature cream cheese.

Sesame Nori Salad Dressing

Imperial (Metric)	American
1 sheet of nori	1 sheet of nori
3 tablespoons roasted sesame seeds	3 tablespoons roasted sesame seeds
4 tablespoons brown rice vinegar	4 tablespoons brown rice vinegar
8 fl oz (230ml) water	1 cup water
½ teaspoon shoyu	½ teaspoon shoyu

1. Toast the sheet of nori by holding it shiny side up horizontally 10 inches (25cm) above a gas flame and rotating it for 3-5 seconds until its colour changes to bright green.
2. Crush the toasted nori into very small pieces.
3. Grind the roasted sesame seeds into a suribachi until 80 per cent ground.
4. Combine all the ingredients and serve as a dressing on grain and noodle salads, boiled and pressed vegetable salads.

Nori Condiment with Sheet Nori

Imperial (Metric)	American
4 fl oz (115ml) water	½ cup water
4 sheets of nori	4 sheets of nori
1 tablespoon shoyu	1 tablespoon shoyu

1. Place the water in a pot, break the nori sheets by hand into small pieces and add to the water. Leave to soak for 10 minutes.
2. Bring to the boil, reduce the heat and simmer for 5 minutes. Add the shoyu and continue to simmer for 2-3 more minutes until the liquid has become absorbed and the nori becomes like a thick paste.

Variation: 1 tablespoon of brown rice vinegar or ½ tablespoon of juice from freshly grated ginger can also be added with the shoyu. Nori Condiment makes an attractive accompaniment to cereal grain dishes.

French Onion Soup with Wild Nori

Serves 3-4

Imperial (Metric)

- 2 pints (1.1 litres) water
- 1 oz (30g) wild nori, soaked 3-4 minutes, chopped finely
- Few drops of sesame oil
- 2 medium onions, cut into fine half moons
- 4 tablespoons shoyu
- 4 oz (115g) breadcrumbs, dried in the oven until crisp, or deep fried
- Chopped parsley to garnish

American

- 5 cups water
- 1 cup wild nori, soaked 3-4 minutes, chopped finely
- Few drops of sesame oil
- 2 medium onions, cut into fine half moons
- 4 tablespoons shoyu
- 1 cup breadcrumbs, dried in the oven until crisp, or deep fried
- Chopped parsley to garnish

1. Place the wild nori together with its soaking water in a pot with the water. Bring to the boil and simmer for 15 minutes.
2. Lightly oil a frying pan and heat. Add the onions and a few drops of shoyu and cook slowly for 50 minutes, adding water as necessary.
3. Add the onions to the soup, season with the remaining shoyu and gently simmer for 3-4 more minutes.
4. Serve the soup garnished with the breadcrumbs and chopped parsley.

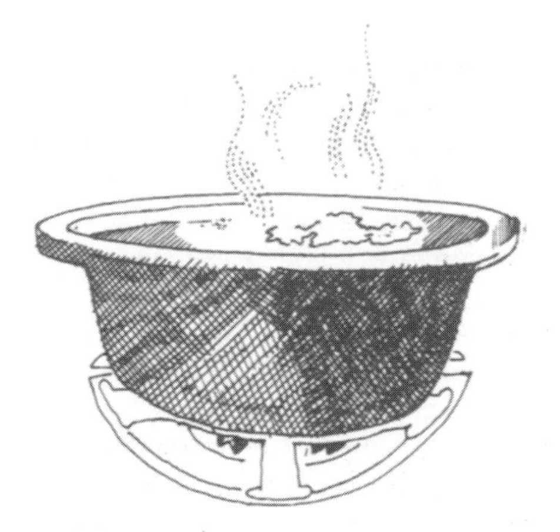

Cold Noodles with Shredded Nori (Zaru Soba)

Serves 3-4

Imperial (Metric)

- 1 packet soba, buckwheat spaghetti*
- 1 strip of kombu, 6 inches (15cm) long
- 2 pints (1.1 litres) water
- 4 tablespoons shoyu
- ½ oz (15g) shredded nori (kizami nori)
- 1 oz (30g) chopped spring onions
- 4 tablespoons roasted sesame seeds
- 2 tablespoons paste prepared from wasabi powder with a few drops water (optional)**

American

- 1 package soba, buckwheat noodles*
- 1 strip of kombu, 6 inches long
- 5 cups water
- 4 tablespoons shoyu
- ½ cup shredded nori (kizami nori)
- ¼ cup chopped scallions
- 4 tablespoons roasted sesame seeds
- 2 tablespoons paste prepared from wasabi powder with a few drops water (optional)**

1. Bring a pot of water to the boil and add the soba. Return to the boil, reduce the heat to medium low and cook until they are done (when a noodle cut in half shows the same colour on both the inside and outside). Place the soba in a strainer, rinse under cold water to prevent sticking and leave to drain.
2. To prepare the dip sauce, place the kombu in a pan with the water. Bring to the boil, simmer for 30 minutes, add the shoyu and simmer for 2-3 minutes more.
3. To serve, place the soba in individual serving bowls with a little kizami nori on top. Serve the dip sauce in smaller individual bowls. Place the spring onions (scallions), the rest of the kizami nori, sesame seeds and wasabi carefully separated again in individual serving dishes for each person.
4. To eat, each person takes a little wasabi to taste from their dish and stirs this into their dip sauce. They then add the spring onions (scallions), roasted sesame seeds and kizami nori to this. They then pick up some soba, dip it in their sauce and eat.

* The standard packet weight is 250g in the UK and Europe, and 8 oz in the USA. Either size could be used in this recipe.

** Natural grated horseradish or ginger can be used instead of wasabi.

Note: Zaru Soba is a delightfully social dish for a group of people and is refreshing, yet sustaining, on a hot day. The set of dishes for each person is usually served on a tray. By having their own set of seasonings each person can adjust the taste of their dip sauce to their own preferences.

Country Style Soup with Wild Nori

Serves 5-6

Imperial (Metric)	American
2½ pints (1.4 litres) water	6¼ cups water
1 oz (30g) wild nori, soaked in 8 fl oz (230ml) water for 3 minutes, finely chopped	1 cup wild nori, soaked in 1 cup water for 3 minutes, finely chopped
4 oz (115g) millet, washed and lightly roasted in a frying pan	½ cup millet, washed and lightly roasted in a skillet
Pinch of sea salt	Pinch of sea salt
5 oz cooked chick peas	1 cup cooked garbanzo beans
3 oz (85g) carrots, diced	½ cup carrots, diced
2 oz (55g) leeks, finely sliced diagonally	1 cup leeks, finely sliced diagonally
1½ tablespoons barley (mugi) miso	1½ tablespoons barley (mugi) miso
Watercress, chopped to garnish	Watercress, chopped to garnish

1. Bring the water and the soaking water from the wild nori to the boil, add the millet and a pinch of sea salt, cover and cook gently for 20 minutes.
2. Add the cooked chick peas (garbanzo beans), wild nori and carrots and cook for 15 minutes.
3. Add the leeks and cook for a further 5 minutes.
4. Mix the miso with a small quantity of the soup liquid, add to the soup and simmer gently for 2-3 minutes.
5. Serve garnished with chopped watercress.

Note: This soup can be prepared with different grains, beans and vegetables. It is a very warming dish for cold days.

Noodles in Broth with Tempura and Wild Nori (Soba Tempura)

Serves 3-4

Imperial (Metric)
1 packet soba, buckwheat spaghetti*
2 pints (1.1 litres) water, for broth
1 oz (30g) wild nori, soaked 3-4 minutes, chopped
1 medium onion, cut into fine half moons
3-4 tablespoons shoyu
2 tablespoons juice from freshly grated ginger
2 spring onions, finely chopped for garnish

Tempura:
2 oz (55g) wholemeal pastry flour
3 tablespoons arrowroot
Pinch of sea salt
4 tablespoons sparkling water or beer
1 medium carrot, cut in matchsticks
Vegetable oil (ideally sesame oil) for deep frying

American
1 package soba, buckwheat noodles*
5 cups water, for broth
1 cup wild nori, soaked 3-4 minutes, chopped
1 medium onion, cut into fine half moons
3-4 tablespoons shoyu
2 tablespoons juice from freshly grated ginger
2 scallions, finely chopped for garnish

Tempura:
½ cup wholewheat pastry flour
3 tablespoons arrowroot
Pinch of sea salt
4 tablespoons sparkling water or beer
1 medium carrot, cut in matchsticks
Vegetable oil (ideally sesame oil) for deep frying

1. Bring a pot of water to the boil, add the soba and bring the water back to the boil. Reduce the heat and cook until done (cut a noodle in half and check the outside colour is the same as the inside colour). Place the soba in a strainer and rinse under cold water to prevent sticking.

2. Place the water for the broth in a pan, add the nori and soaking water, bring to the boil, add the onions and cook uncovered for 10 minutes. Add the shoyu and ginger juice and simmer for 2 minutes.

3. Prepare the tempura batter by combining the wholemeal flour, arrowroot, and a pinch of sea salt in a bowl. Gradually add the

sparkling water or beer to make a thick batter. Leave to stand at least half an hour in the refrigerator to produce a crispier tempura. Add the carrot matchsticks and mix well.

4. Heat the oil (at least 2-3 inches deep) for deep frying to 350°F/180°C. Do not let it smoke. Drop in a small piece of the batter to check the temperature. It should sink to the bottom and then rise quickly to the surface.
5. Deep fry the tempura batter in spoonsful, turning each piece until it is golden brown all over. Remove and drain on a paper towel.
6. Add the cooked noodles to the broth and warm for a few minutes.
7. In a large bowl for each person, add the noodles and broth and place a few pieces of tempura on top. Garnish with the chopped spring onions (scallions).

* The standard weight of a packet is 250g in the UK and Europe, and 8 oz in the USA. Either size could be used in this recipe.

Note: Sparkling mineral water or beer work like egg in giving a light and crunchy texture to the tempura.

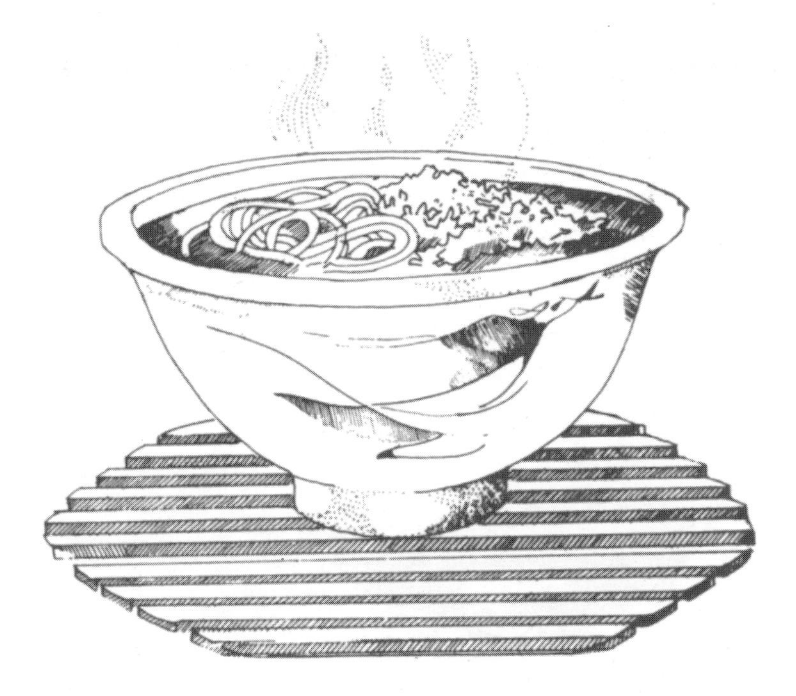

Fried Rice with Wild Nori

Serves 3-4

Imperial (Metric)	American
Sesame oil (preferably roasted)	Sesame oil (preferably roasted)
6 oz (170g) onions, diced	1 cup onions, diced
2 oz (55g) carrots, cut into matchsticks	½ cup carrots, cut into matchsticks
1 oz (30g) wild nori, soaked 3-4 minutes, chopped finely	1 cup wild nori, soaked 3-4 minutes, chopped finely
2 oz (55g) celery, diced	½ cup celery, diced
2 tablespoons shoyu	2 tablespoons shoyu
¾ lb (340g) cooked brown rice	2 cups cooked brown rice
2 tablespoons juice from freshly grated ginger root	2 tablespoons juice from freshly grated ginger root
2 oz (55g) chopped roasted almonds	½ cup chopped roasted almonds

1. Lightly oil a frying pan and heat. Add the onions and sauté uncovered for 5-7 minutes. Add the carrots and wild nori and cook for 5-7 minutes. Add the celery and 1 tablespoon of the shoyu and cook for a further 5 minutes.
2. Add the cooked brown rice, 3-4 tablespoons of the soaking water from the wild nori, 1 more tablespoon shoyu and the ginger juice and mix well. Gently stir continuously for 2-3 minutes.
3. Add the chopped roasted almonds and serve.

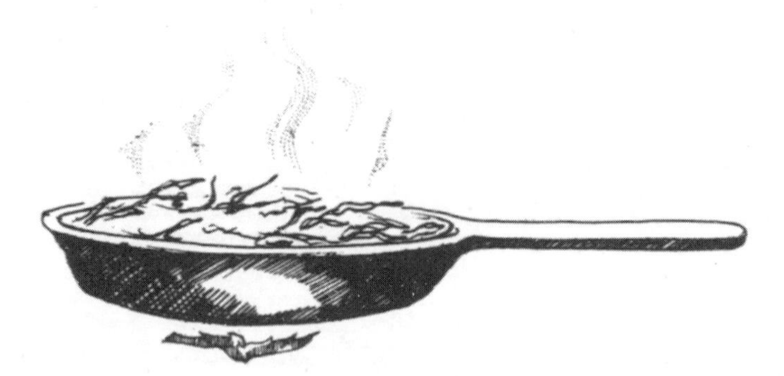

Tempeh Stew with Wild Nori

Serves 4-5

Imperial (Metric)	American
½ lb (225g) block of tempeh	½ pound block of tempeh
Sesame oil for deep frying	Sesame oil for deep frying
2 oz (55g) wild nori, soaked 3-4 minutes, chopped	2 cups wild nori, soaked 3-4 minutes, chopped
¾ pint (425ml) water	2 cups water
2 tablespoons shoyu	2 tablespoons shoyu
2 medium turnips, quartered	2 medium turnips, quartered
9 oz (255g) pumpkin, seeds removed, cut into 1 inch by 1½ inch (2.5 × 4cm) cubes	1½ cups winter squash, seeds removed, cut into 1 inch by 1½ inch cubes
4 oz (115g) leeks, cut diagonally in 2 inch (5cm) lengths	1 cup leeks, cut diagonally in 2 inch lengths

1. If the tempeh has been deep frozen allow time for it to thoroughly thaw out before using. Cut into 1 inch (2.5cm) squares.
2. Heat 2-3 inches of the sesame oil in a pan to 350°F/180°C. Make sure it does not smoke.
3. Deep fry the tempeh squares for 3-4 minutes until their colour changes. Remove from the oil and leave to drain on a paper towel.
4. Place the wild nori together with its soaking water in a heavy pan. Add the fried tempeh, the water and 1 tablespoon of the shoyu and cook, covered, over a medium heat for 10 minutes.
5. Add the turnips, pumpkin (squash) and the remaining tablespoon of shoyu and cook for 10 minutes.
6. Add the leeks and cook for a further 10 minutes or until the liquid has completely evaporated.

Note: Each vegetable is added at a different stage to give the right amount of cooking by the end of the preparation.

Stuffed Cabbage Leaves with Wild Nori

Serves 3-4

Imperial (Metric)

6 white cabbage leaves
Pinch of sea salt
Few drops of sesame oil
6 oz (170g) onions, diced
1 oz (30g) burdock, diced
1 oz (30g) wild nori, soaked 3-4 minutes, finely chopped
6 shiitake mushrooms, soaked 10 minutes, finely sliced
6 oz (170g) tofu, crushed with a fork
2 tablespoons shoyu
12 cocktail sticks

American

6 white cabbage leaves
Pinch of sea salt
Few drops of sesame oil
1 cup onions, diced
¼ cup burdock, diced
1 cup wild nori, soaked 3-4 minutes, finely chopped
6 shiitake mushrooms, soaked 10 minutes, finely sliced
1 cup tofu, crushed with a fork
2 tablespoons shoyu
12 cocktail sticks

1. Boil the cabbage leaves for 2-3 minutes in a pan of water with a pinch of sea salt. Remove, and place on a plate to cool.
2. Lightly oil a frying pan and heat. Sauté the onions uncovered for 5-7 minutes, then add the burdock and sauté for a further 5-7 minutes.

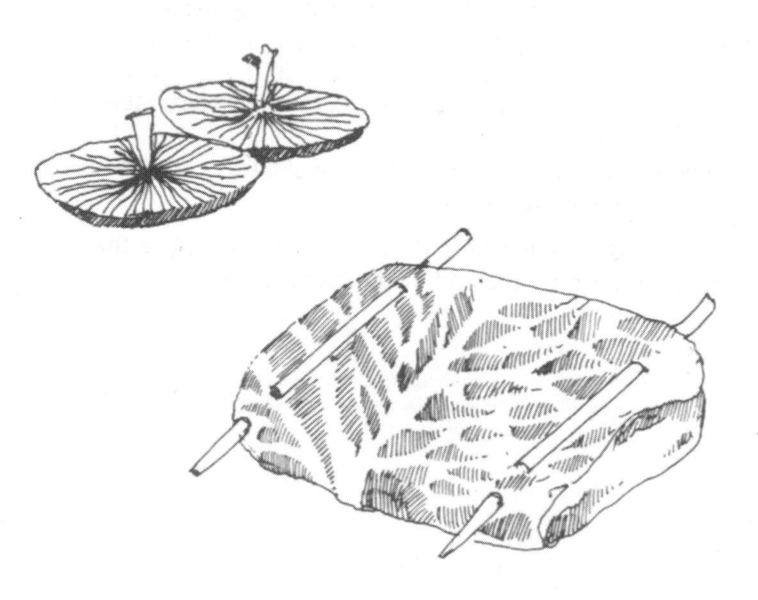

3. Add the wild nori, shiitake mushrooms, tofu and shoyu. Cover and simmer gently for a further 10 minutes, adding a small amount of the soaking water if necessary.
4. Place one cabbage leaf at a time on a cutting board. Lay flat and put 2-3 tablespoons of the cooked vegetables in the middle. Neatly roll up the leaf, securing each end by pinning through with a cocktail stick.
5. Arrange attractively on a serving plate.

Note: These cabbage rolls can be served with a hot sauce made with ¾ pint/425ml (2 cups) water, 1 tablespoon shoyu, 1 tablespoon fresh ginger juice and 1 tablespoon kuzu diluted in ⅔ pint/340ml (1½ cups) of cold water. Mix the ingredients together in a pan and cook for ½-1 minute, stirring constantly, until thick and clear.

Wild Nori Condiment

Imperial (Metric)	American
Few drops of sesame oil	Few drops of sesame oil
1 medium carrot, finely chopped	1 medium carrot, finely chopped
1 oz (30g) wild nori, soaked for 3 minutes, chopped finely	1 cup wild nori, soaked for 3 minutes, chopped finely
1 bunch spring onions, finely chopped	1 bunch scallions, finely chopped
4 tablespoons brown rice (genmai) miso, diluted with 3 tablespoons soaking water from the nori	4 tablespoons brown rice (genmai) miso, diluted with 3 tablespoons soaking water from the nori
2 tablespoons juice from freshly grated ginger root	2 tablespoons juice from freshly grated ginger root

1. Lightly oil a frying pan and heat. Add the carrot and sauté for 5-7 minutes. Add the nori and spring onions (scallions) and sauté for 5 more minutes.
2. Add the diluted miso and ginger juice. Cover and simmer gently for 5 minutes or until the liquid has completely evaporated.
3. Serve on cereal grains or as a small side dish with a meal.

Note: A powdered nori condiment can be made by roasting wild nori in an oven at 375°F/190°C (Gas Mark 5) until it becomes crisp, and then grinding to a fine powder in a suribachi. It can also be ground with roasted seeds.

Mochi (Pounded Sweet Rice) with Green Nori Flakes

Serves 8

Imperial (Metric)	American
1 lb (450g) sweet brown rice	2 cups sweet brown rice
1 pint (570ml) water	2½ cups water
Pinch of sea salt	Pinch of sea salt
¾ oz (20g) green nori flakes	1 cup green nori flakes

1. Rinse the rice and put in a pressure cooker with the water and a pinch of sea salt. Allow the pressure to come up fully, reduce the heat to low and cook for 45 minutes. Turn off the heat and allow the pressure to reduce naturally.
2. Place the rice in a large, heavy wooden bowl and with a wooden pestle pound it vigorously for about 20 minutes or until all the grains are broken and the texture becomes very sticky. Wet the pestle occasionally or sprinkle a little water on the rice to make the pounding easier.
3. Wet your hands and form small balls of the pounded rice (mochi). With dry hands roll these in a bowl containing the green nori flakes. (The best technique, which requires a little practice, is to have one wet hand for forming the balls, and the other hand dry for rolling.)

Note: These mochi balls (Nori Ohagi) make a very attractive party food or snack and are ideal for picnics or travelling. They can also be rolled in roasted black or white sesame seeds and a combination of coatings makes a most attractive dish. Pounded sweet rice (mochi) is a very sustaining food and especially popular during winter.

Crêpes with Green Nori Flakes

Imperial (Metric)	American
4 oz (115g) wholemeal pastry flour	1 cup wholewheat pastry flour
1 pint (570ml) water (approx)	2½ cups water (approx)
Pinch of sea salt	Pinch of sea salt
½ oz (15g) green nori flakes	½ cup green nori flakes
Sesame oil	Sesame oil

Please send us this card to receive our latest catalog.

❐ Check here if you would like to receive our catalog via e-mail.

E-mail address ______________________________

Name ____________________ Company ____________________

Address ______________________________ Phone ______________

City ____________________ State ______ Zip ________ Country __________

Please check the following area(s) of interest to you:

❐ Health ❐ Self-help ❐ Spirituality ❐ Shamanism
❐ Ancient Mysteries ❐ New Age ❐ Tarot ❐ Martial Arts
❐ Spanish Language ❐ Sexuality/Drugs ❐ Children ❐ Teen

Order at 1-800-246-8648 • Fax (802) 767-3726
E-mail: orders@InnerTraditions.com • Web site: www.InnerTraditions.com

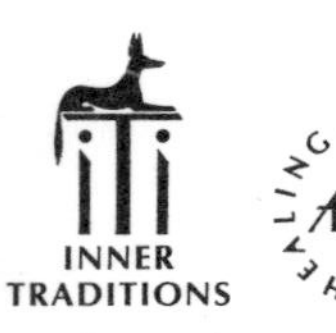

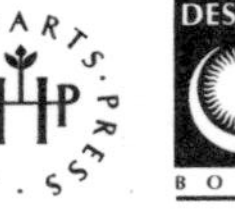

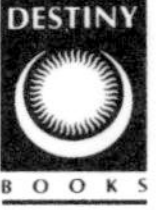

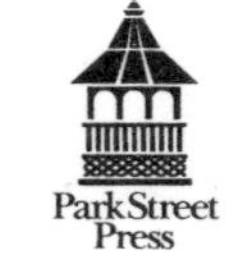

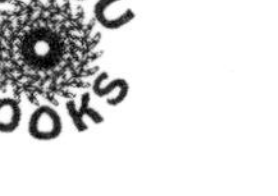

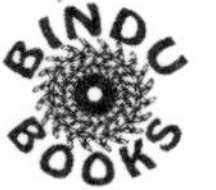
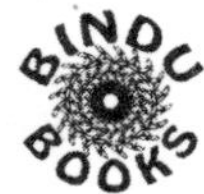

Affix
Postage
Stamp
Here

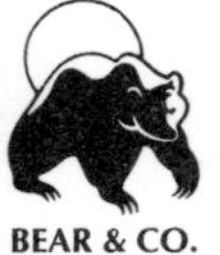

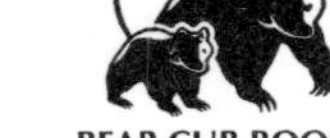

Inner Traditions • Bear & Company
P.O. Box 388
Rochester, VT 05767-0388
U.S.A.

1. Beat the water into the flour in a mixing bowl to form a very thin batter. The amount of water used may vary, as different flours can have different absorbencies. Add a pinch of sea salt with the green nori flakes, mix again and set aside for 30 minutes.
2. Brush a small amount of sesame oil on a flat frying pan or crêpe pan. Heat and pour on a small amount of the batter to evenly cover the surface tilting the pan to form a round shape. Cook one side of the crêpe then flip over and briefly cook the other side. Remove crêpe, put on a large plate and cover with a cloth to keep soft. Repeat the process, making as many crêpes as desired.
3. To fill the crêpes, spread 2 tablespoons of your chosen filling (see pages 55-56) across each crêpe, roll and serve.

Note: Green nori flakes make an attractive ingredient in a crêpe batter. They are suitable for either savoury or sweet fillings. The two key factors in making good crêpes are firstly a smooth batter of the right consistency, and secondly, having the pan at just the right temperature. A little practice will produce a satisfactory crêpe without resorting to using eggs or binding agents.

Sesame Daikon Savoury Filling

Imperial (Metric)	American
3 oz (85g) grated daikon radish	½ cup grated daikon radish
1 tablespoon sesame spread	1 tablespoon sesame butter
1 teaspoon shoyu	1 teaspoon shoyu
2 tablespoons water	2 tablespoons water

1. Combine all the ingredients in a suribachi and mix well until the sesame spread (sesame butter) has dissolved.

Tofu Watercress Savoury Filling

Imperial (Metric)	American
½ lb (225g) block of tofu	½ pound block of tofu
½ bunch watercress, chopped	½ bunch watercress, chopped
2 tablespoons umeboshi vinegar	2 tablespoons umeboshi vinegar

1. Boil the tofu for five minutes, then mash in a suribachi.
2. Add the chopped watercress and umeboshi vinegar and mix well.

Carrot Mustard Savoury Filling

Imperial (Metric)	American
4 oz (115g) carrot, grated	1 cup carrot, grated
2 tablespoons natural mustard	2 tablespoons natural mustard
1 teaspoon shoyu	1 teaspoon shoyu
1 tablespoon water	1 tablespoon water

1. Combine all the ingredients and mix well.

Apple Walnut Sweet Filling

Imperial (Metric)	American
3 apples, cut into small pieces	3 apples, cut into small pieces
3 tablespoons barley malt	3 tablespoons barley malt
Pinch of sea salt	Pinch of sea salt
8 fl oz (230ml) water	1 cup water
1 tablespoon kuzu, diluted in 2 tablespoons cold water	1 tablespoon kuzu, diluted in 2 tablespoons cold water
2 oz (55g) chopped roasted walnuts	½ cup chopped roasted walnuts

1. Place the apples, a pinch of sea salt and the water in a pan, bring to the boil and simmer for 10-15 minutes.
2. Add the barley malt and stir in.
3. Add the diluted kuzu and stir gently for ½-1 minute to obtain a thick and clear consistency. Add the chopped roasted walnuts.

Apricot Orange Sweet Filling

Imperial (Metric)	American
10 oz (285g) dried apricots	2 cups dried apricots
1½ pints (850ml) water	3¾ cups water
Pinch of sea salt	Pinch of sea salt
1½ tablespoons orange rind, grated	1½ tablespoons orange rind, grated
1 tablespoon kuzu, diluted in 2 tablespoons cold water	1 tablespoon kuzu, diluted in 2 tablespoons cold water

1. Wash the apricots thoroughly. Soak in the water for 2-3 hours.
2. Bring to the boil with a pinch of sea salt and the grated orange rind and simmer for 30 minutes.

3. Add the diluted kuzu and stir gently for ½-1 minute to obtain a thick and clear consistency.

Sesame Daikon Sauce with Green Nori Flakes

Imperial (Metric)	American
4 tablespoons boiling water	4 tablespoons boiling water
2 tablespoons sesame spread	2 tablespoons sesame butter
4 oz (115g) grated daikon radish	1 cup grated daikon radish
3 tablespoons green nori flakes	3 tablespoons green nori flakes
1 tablespoon umeboshi vinegar	1 tablespoon umeboshi vinegar
½ teaspoon shoyu	½ teaspoon shoyu

1. Mix the boiling water with the sesame spread (sesame butter) to make a smooth cream.
2. Add all the other ingredients and mix together.

Note: More or less water can be used to create a thinner or thicker sauce as desired. This sauce combines well with deep-fried dishes and is an ideal topping for fried or baked mochi (see page 54).

Tofu Dip with Green Nori Flakes

Imperial (Metric)	American
6 oz (170g) tofu	1 cup tofu
4 fl oz (115ml) water	½ cup water
1½ tablespoons barley (mugi) miso	1½ tablespoons barley (mugi) miso
4 fl oz (115ml) liquid from pickles, or brown rice vinegar, or orange juice	½ cup liquid from pickles, or brown rice vinegar, or orange juice
⅓ oz (10g) green nori flakes	½ cup green nori flakes

1. Crumble the tofu by hand, then place in a suribachi and blend until it forms a creamy consistency.
2. Heat the water and dilute the miso in it. Add to the tofu.
3. Add the remaining ingredients and mix well.

Note: This dip is very popular at parties and can be served with crackers or used as a spread for sandwiches. The use of green nori flakes is an attractive alternative to the more common use of chives.

Marinated Salad with Purple Leaf Nori (Fu-Nori)

Serves 2-3

Imperial (Metric)	American
½ oz (15g) fu-nori	1 cup fu-nori
½ a cucumber	½ a cucumber
Pinch of sea salt	Pinch of sea salt
2 fl oz (60ml) water	¼ cup water
4 fl oz (115ml) brown rice vinegar	½ cup brown rice vinegar
3 tablespoons shoyu	3 tablespoons shoyu
3 oz (85g) fresh mushrooms, cut finely	1 cup fresh mushrooms, cut finely

1. Rinse the fu-nori quickly, soak for 30 seconds and squeeze out excess liquid.
2. Cut the cucumber lengthwise and slice diagonally into half moons. Sprinkle with a few grains of sea salt and leave for 1 hour, mixing occasionally. Squeeze gently, discarding the excess liquid, then add to the fu-nori.
3. Put the water, brown rice vinegar, shoyu and mushrooms into a saucepan. Bring to the boil, reduce the heat to medium and cook uncovered for 10-15 minutes until all the liquid has evaporated.
4. Allow to cool and then mix with the cucumber and the fu-nori.

Note: If the seasoning is not strong enough, add a small amount of brown rice vinegar to the finished salad. Fu-nori can be used in many ways for soups, salads, condiments and garnishes.

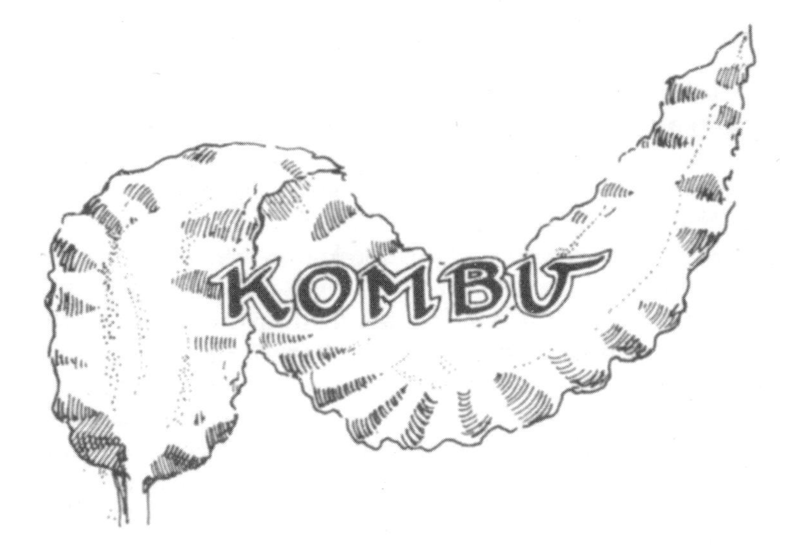

Thick dark strips of kombu are an essential cooking ingredient. It can be used as a flavouring, a natural sweetener, and a softening agent, as well as being cooked as a vegetable in its own right. Kombu, often known as kelp in the West, describes a wide range of brown sea vegetables, mostly from the *laminaria* family, that grow abundantly just below the tide line. They vary considerably in form but generally all have broad, smooth and shiny fronds. They have been used since antiquity not only in the Far East, but also around Atlantic shores where they are known by various names including *wrack*, *tangle* and *oarweed*.

Kombu is rich in alginic acid, the strong binding agent that holds the plant structure together and keeps it flexible enough to withstand the constant pounding surf of its natural habitat. This alginic acid, because of its indigestible nature and binding quality, acts as a natural cleanser for the intestines by gathering together the toxins within the colon wall and allowing for their natural elimination. Kombu also strengthens the intestines, and a traditional recipe from Japan, known as *shio-kombu*, has been used for centuries as a remedy for colitis. It is prepared by soaking kombu, cutting into small squares, and cooking down with shoyu and water until soft and the liquid has disappeared. A few pieces are served with each meal.

Kombu is also rich in glutamic acid, the original natural version of that powerful flavouring agent monosodium glutamate (MSG), which nowadays is chemically synthesized from molasses. A strip of kombu soaked and cooked briefly with water (long cooking will release stronger tasting mineral salts into the water) will make a delicious stock for soups and noodle broths. This stock, known as *dashi*, is the basis of many a tasty Japanese dish. Its value was recognized long ago by Buddhist monks whose strict laws forbade them to use any ingredient of animal origin. Glutamic acid also has the ability to soften the fibres of other foods. A strip of kombu cooked with beans or dried chestnuts will not only soften them quicker, thereby reducing the cooking time, but will also improve their flavour, add valuable nutrients and increase the overall digestibility of the dish. This softening process works both ways as kombu itself becomes much softer when cooked with protein-rich foods. In addition to sweetness from glutamic acid, kombu contain two simple sugars, fucose and mannitol, which can be of importance to diabetics as they do not raise the blood sugar level.

Kombu is one of the sea vegetables richest in iodine and for centuries the Chinese have used it for the treatment of goitre. In the Far East, where kombu is eaten regularly, there has never been any need to iodize table salt as is commonly done in many western countries. Kombu also contains certain amino acids that act as a gentle stimulant to the mucous membranes and lymphatic system and has long been recognized as a guardian against high blood-pressure, especially amongst the elderly. By promoting the balanced absorption and distribution of nutrients in the body, kombu is beneficial as well to overweight or underweight people by helping to restore their normal weight condition. The health attributes to kombu are so numerous that they can best be summed up in the words of an American scientist who wrote over fifty years ago, 'Of the 14 elements essential to the proper metabolic functions of the human body, 13 are known to be in kelp . . . It should be made available for all people in all lands.'

Kombu is usually sold in the West dried and packaged in strips, but in the Far East it is readily available in numerous forms. We spent one enjoyable afternoon in Japan browsing around a shop that sold nothing but kombu products. There were over 300 items on display that ranged from varying priced strips of kombu, each for a specific cooking use, to many types of cut, shredded and prepared kombu, kombu pickles, condiments, sweets, snacks and teas. Several of these kombu products are now finding their way to the West and can be obtained from a good wholefood store. Some of the most common are:-

Ne-kombu — the mineral-rich holdfast, or root, of kombu. It is very tough and needs long soaking and even longer cooking, but is prized for its rich, sweet, almost liquorice-like flavour. It should be boiled in water seasoned with shoyu until soft and the liquid cooked away, and then served in small portions as a side dish. It is especially strengthening for the intestines.

Shredded (nalto)-kombu — strip kombu cut into thin strands. It can be used for a quick dashi stock, or added to soups, or simply prepared as a vegetable.

Instant (tororo) kombu — a selected grade of kombu that has been sun-dried, soaked in mild rice vinegar for several days, and then shaved into thin hair-like threads. It needs virtually no cooking. Either add to soups at the end of cooking, or soften with boiling water and a dash of shoyu and serve as a side dish. Its delightfully sweet, yet mildly sour taste will add a refreshing piquancy to your meal.

Kombu powder (kombu-ko) — premium quality kombu that has been dried and simply ground into a very fine powder. It has an appealing sweet flavour and can be sprinkled on food as a condiment or cooked in water to prepare a nutritious drink.

Kelp powder as marketed by the health food industry is usually ground from ungraded Atlantic varieties of kombu and has a coarse texture with a stronger sea flavour than Japanese kombu powder. It is sometimes used as a food supplement but we find that it also makes an excellent tonic to add to bath water.

Clear Kombu Soup

Serves 2-3

Imperial (Metric)

1 6-inch (15cm) long strip of kombu
1½ pints (850ml) water
1 small piece each of carrot, radish and turnip, finely cut
4 teaspoons shoyu
Spring onions, parsley or watercress, finely cut to garnish

American

1 6-inch long strip of kombu
3¾ cups of water
1 small piece each of carrot, radish and turnip, finely cut
4 teaspoons shoyu
Scallions, parsley or watercress, finely cut, to garnish

1. If the kombu is dusty or covered with white powder, wipe clean with a damp cloth.
2. Place the kombu in a pot, add the water and bring to the boil. Simmer for 10-15 minutes.
3. Remove the kombu and place on a mat to dry, saving to use again.
4. Add a small amount of finely cut vegetables to the water and cook for 5 minutes.
5. Season with the shoyu and garnish with either finely cut spring onions (scallions), parsley or watercress.

Note: If you prefer a stronger flavour, leave the kombu to simmer longer.

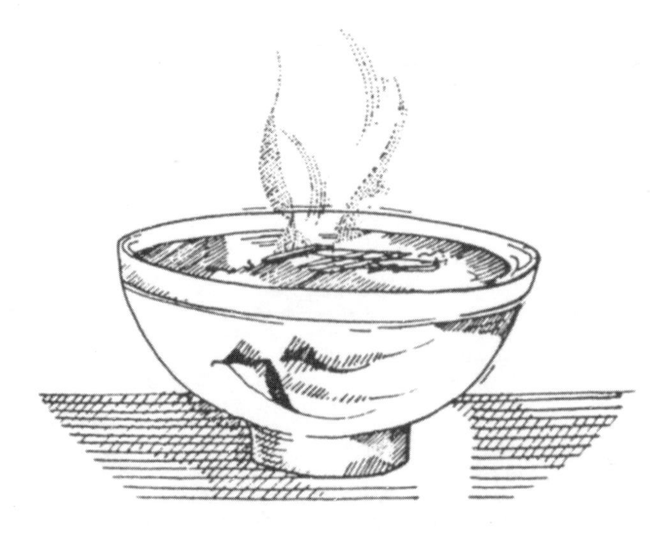

Barley Casserole

Serves 3-4

Imperial (Metric)

½ lb (225g) pot or pearled barley
1¼ pints (700ml) water
1 6-inch (15cm) strip of kombu
6 oz (170g) onions, diced
3 oz (85g) pumpkin, diced
1½ oz (45g) burdock, cut into fine matchsticks (optional)
1½ oz (45g) seitan wheat gluten, diced
Pinch of sea salt
Parsley, chopped to garnish

American

1 cup pot or pearled barley
3 cups water
1 6-inch strip of kombu
1 cup onions, diced
½ cup pumpkin, diced
¼ cup burdock, cut into fine matchsticks (optional)
¼ cup seitan wheat meat, diced
Pinch of sea salt
Parsley, chopped to garnish

1. Wash the barley and soak for 5 hours in the water. Wipe the kombu clean with a damp cloth and soak with the barley for ½ hour. Remove and cut into thin strips.
2. Put the soaking water from the barley into a pressure cooker and bring to the boil. Add the onions and cook for 3 minutes without the lid.
3. Place the other vegetables and the kombu, seitan and barley in layers in the pot. Add a pinch of sea salt.
4. Bring to a high pressure, reduce the heat and cook for 45 minutes. Turn off the heat, let the pressure reduce naturally, open and transfer to a serving bowl.
5. Garnish with the chopped parsley.

Lentil Stew

Serves 4-5

Imperial (Metric)
6 oz (170g) lentils
1 6-inch (15cm) long strip of kombu
1½ pints (850ml) water
6 oz (170g) onions, chopped
3 oz (85g) carrots, chopped
3 oz (85g) celery, chopped
¼ teaspoon sea salt
Spring onions, chopped to garnish

American
1 cup lentils
1 6-inch long strip of kombu
3¾ cups water
1 cup onions, chopped
½ cup carrots, chopped
½ cup celery, chopped
¼ teaspoon sea salt
Scallions, chopped to garnish

1. Place the lentils a handful at a time on a plate and sort out any small stones.
2. Wash the lentils and place in a pot with the kombu on the bottom and add the water. Bring to the boil, reduce the heat to low, cover and simmer for about one hour or until they are almost soft.
3. Add the onions and cook uncovered for 5 minutes.
4. Add the carrots, celery and sea salt, cover and cook for a further 10-15 minutes. Check during cooking that there is sufficient water, adding more if necessary.
5. Remove the lid, turn the heat up to medium and boil off the excess water.

Note: Cooking kombu with beans reduces the cooking time, helps soften the beans and also makes them more digestible.

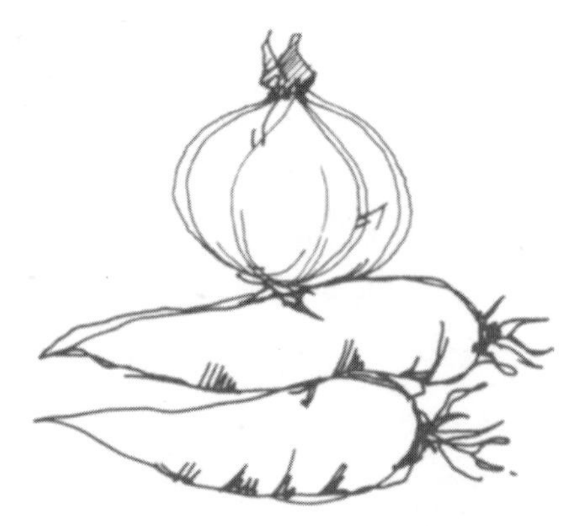

Hummus

Serves 3-4

Imperial (Metric)	American
½ lb (225g) chick peas	1 cup garbanzo beans
1¼ pints (700ml) water	3 cups water
1 5-inch (12.5cm) strip of kombu	1 5-inch strip of kombu
¼ teaspoon sea salt	¼ teaspoon sea salt
2 cloves garlic, peeled and finely chopped	2 cloves garlic, peeled and finely chopped
Juice of 2 lemons	Juice of 2 lemons
1 tablespoon umeboshi vinegar	1 tablespoon umeboshi vinegar
2 tablespoons tahini	2 tablespoons tahini

1. Spread the chick peas (garbanzo beans) on a plate and carefully sort out any stones.
2. Soak the chick peas (garbanzo beans) overnight.
3. Place the chick peas (garbanzo beans) in a pressure cooker discarding the soaking water. Add 1¼ pints/700ml (3 cups) fresh water and the kombu and pressure cook for 1½ hours.
4. Remove from heat, open, add the sea salt and then pressure cook again for 20 minutes.
5. Purée the chick peas (garbanzo beans), kombu and any remaining liquid with the other ingredients in a blender. If the consistency is too thick, add some water.
6. To store, keep in a refrigerator.

Note: Salt inhibits the softening of beans during cooking which is why it is added towards the end. Kombu, on the other hand, aids their softening.

Sweet and Sour Tempeh

Serves 3-4

Imperial (Metric)	American
½ lb (225g) block of tempeh	½ pound block of tempeh
Vegetable oil for deep frying (preferably unrefined sesame oil)	Vegetable oil for deep frying (preferably unrefined sesame oil)
2 5-inch (12.5cm) strips of kombu	2 5-inch strips of kombu
8 fl oz (230ml) water	1 cup water
4 medium carrots, cut into chunks	4 medium carrots, cut into chunks
3 tablespoons shoyu	3 tablespoons shoyu
2 tablespoons mirin or barley malt	2 tablespoons mirin or barley malt
3 tablespoons brown rice vinegar	3 tablespoons brown rice vinegar
Spring onions, chopped to garnish	Scallions, chopped to garnish

1. If the tempeh has been deep frozen allow time to thoroughly thaw out before using.
2. Cut the tempeh into rectangles about 1½ inches × 3 inches (4cm × 7.5cm).
3. Heat the oil in a deep frying pan to 350°F/180°C. Deep fry the tempeh for 2 or 3 minutes until the colour changes. Remove from the oil and drain on a paper towel.
4. Place the kombu in the bottom of a heavy pot, cover with the water and soak for 1 hour. Cut the kombu into fine strips and return to the pot.
5. Add the fried tempeh, carrots, shoyu, mirin or barley malt, brown rice vinegar and any additional water needed to cover the tempeh. Cook for 20 minutes on a medium heat or until the liquid has evaporated.
6. Garnish with the chopped spring onions (scallions).

Daikon with Half Moon Orange Sauce

Serves 3-4

Imperial (Metric)	American
1 6-inch (15cm) strip of kombu	1 6-inch strip of kombu
8 fl oz (230ml) water	1 cup water
1 medium daikon radish, cut into rounds ½ inch (1cm) thick	1 medium daikon radish, cut into rounds ½ inch thick
Sauce:	*Sauce:*
3 oz (85g) roasted sesame seeds	½ cup roasted sesame seeds
2 tablespoons grated orange rind	2 tablespoons grated orange rind
1 tablespoon barley (mugi) miso	1 tablespoon barley (mugi) miso
6 tablespoons water	6 tablespoons water

1. In a pot, soak the kombu with the water for 1 hour. Add the daikon rounds and bring to the boil. Reduce the flame to medium, cover and cook for 10-15 minutes. Remove the daikon rounds and arrange on a serving plate with each piece lying flat.
2. Prepare the sauce by grinding the roasted sesame seeds in a suribachi until they are powdered. Add the remaining sauce ingredients and mix well to obtain a smooth creamy sauce.
3. Place a small amount of the sauce on top of each daikon round forming a half moon shape.
4. Serve warm or cold as desired.

Note: The kombu is not actually used in serving this dish and can be kept for use in another recipe.

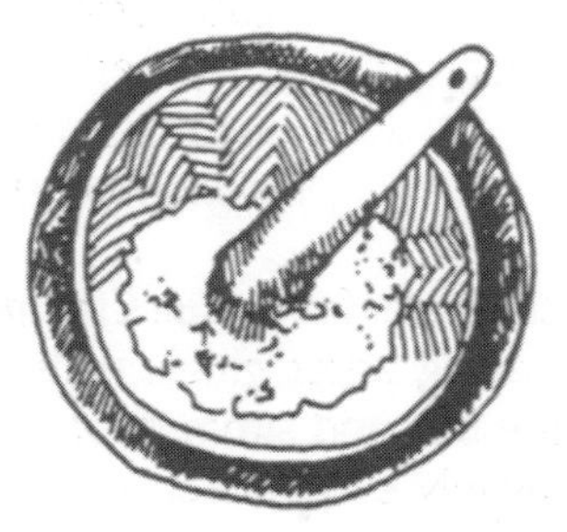

Carrot Kombu Rolls

Serves 2

Imperial (Metric)	American
4 strips of kombu, each 8 inches (20cm) long	4 strips of kombu, each 8 inches long
¾ pint (425ml) water	2 cups water
2 medium carrots, cut into 2½ inch (6.5cm) lengths	2 medium carrots, cut into 2½ inch lengths
1 teaspoon shoyu	1 teaspoon shoyu

1. Soak the kombu in the water for 1 hour.
2. Cut 3 of the strips of soaked kombu into 2½ inch (6.5cm) lengths and wrap each one around a piece of carrot. With the fourth strip of soaked kombu, cut it lengthwise into thin strips and tie 1 strip around each kombu covered carrot, securing it with a knot. Alternatively use a cocktail stick.
3. Place the kombu-covered carrots and the soaking water in a pot, bring to the boil and cook covered on a medium heat for 45 minutes. Add the shoyu and cook uncovered for a further 10-15 minutes until all the liquid has evaporated.
4. Remove from the pot and serve the rolls standing on end so the carrot shows.

Kombu Ginger Condiment

Imperial (Metric)	American
2 strips of kombu, each 6 inches (15cm) long	2 strips of kombu, each 6 inches long
8 fl oz (230ml) water	1 cup water
½ oz (45g) fresh ginger root, cut into fine matchsticks	¼ cup fresh ginger root, cut into fine matchsticks
1 tablespoon shoyu	1 tablespoon shoyu

1. Soak the kombu in the water for 1 hour. Cut into very fine strips.
2. Place the kombu, soaking water, ginger matchsticks and shoyu in a pan, bring to the boil and simmer for 35-40 minutes until the liquid has completely evaporated.
3. Serve in very small quantities as a condiment to accompany your meal.

Nishime Root Vegetable Stew

Serves 2-3

Imperial (Metric)
1 6-inch (15cm) long strip of kombu
2 medium carrots, cut into chunks
1 medium parsnip, cut into chunks
Pinch of sea salt
Shoyu to taste

American
1 6-inch long strip of kombu
2 medium carrots, cut into chunks
1 medium parsnip, cut into chunks
Pinch of sea salt
Shoyu to taste

1. Place the kombu in a heavy cooking pot with enough water to cover and soak for 1 hour.
2. Add the vegetables in layers and a pinch of sea salt. Cover and cook over a medium to high heat for 15 to 20 minutes.
3. Add a few drops of shoyu, shake the pot several times to mix the vegetables well, then cook for 2 minutes more or until the liquid has completely evaporated.
4. Remove and cut the kombu into fine strips and serve with the stew.

Note: This is a very strengthening and warming dish, and ideal for serving regularly during winter. Try also with other combinations of root vegetables.

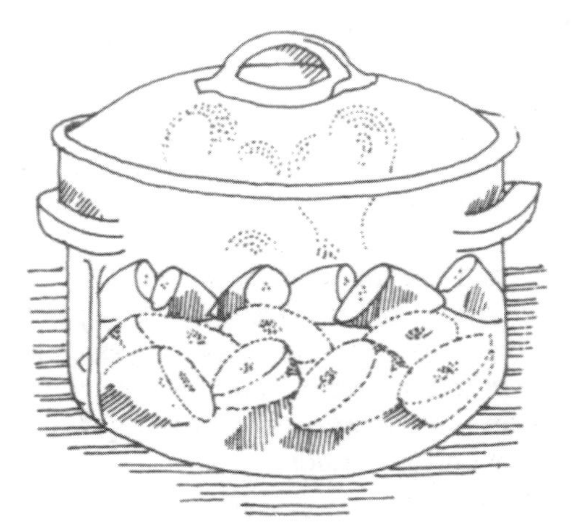

Roasted Kombu Condiment

Imperial (Metric)	American
1 strip of kombu	1 strip of kombu

1. With a damp cloth carefully wipe off any dust or white powder from the kombu.
2. Roast in a moderate oven at 375°F/190°C (Gas Mark 5) for 7-10 minutes until crisp.
3. Grind into a fine powder in a suribachi or mortar and pestle.
4. When cool store in an air-tight jar and use sprinkled sparingly on whole grain dishes. This condiment is very rich in minerals and can be used instead of a normal salty table condiment.

Variation: Mix the kombu powder with roasted and ground sesame, sunflower or pumpkin seeds.

Kombu Salt Pickles

Imperial (Metric)	American
2 teaspoons sea salt	2 teaspoons sea salt
⅔ pint (340ml) water	1½ cups water
1 5-inch (12.5cm) long strip of kombu	1 5-inch long strip of kombu
5 oz (140g) cauliflower, cut into small florets	1 cup cauliflower, cut into small florets
1 medium carrot, cut into thin slices	1 medium carrot, cut into thin slices

1. Combine sea salt and water, bring to the boil and simmer for a few minutes until the salt dissolves. Allow this brine solution to cool.
2. Wash, clean and cut the vegetables.
3. Sprinkle the bottom of a sterilized jar with a pinch of sea salt.
4. Place the kombu and the vegetables in layers in the jar until it is full or the vegetables are used up. (The kombu can either be cut into pieces with scissors or left whole.)
5. Add the cooled brine solution.
6. Keep the jar, uncovered, in a cool place. After 3-4 days the pickles will be ready to eat.
7. To store, cover and refrigerate.

Kombu Shoyu Pickles

Imperial (Metric)
4 fl oz (115ml) shoyu
8 fl oz (230ml) water
1 6-inch (15cm) strip of kombu, cut with scissors into 1 inch (2.5cm) pieces or left whole
9 oz (255g) turnip, cut into thin slices
5 thin slices of fresh ginger root

American
½ cup shoyu
1 cup water
1 6-inch strip of kombu, cut with scissors into 1 inch pieces or left whole
1½ cups turnips, cut into thin slices
5 thin slices of fresh ginger root

1. Combine the shoyu, water, kombu, turnips and ginger in a sterilized jar.
2. Keep the jar uncovered in a cool place.
3. After 3 days the pickles will be ready to eat.
4. To store, cover and refrigerate.

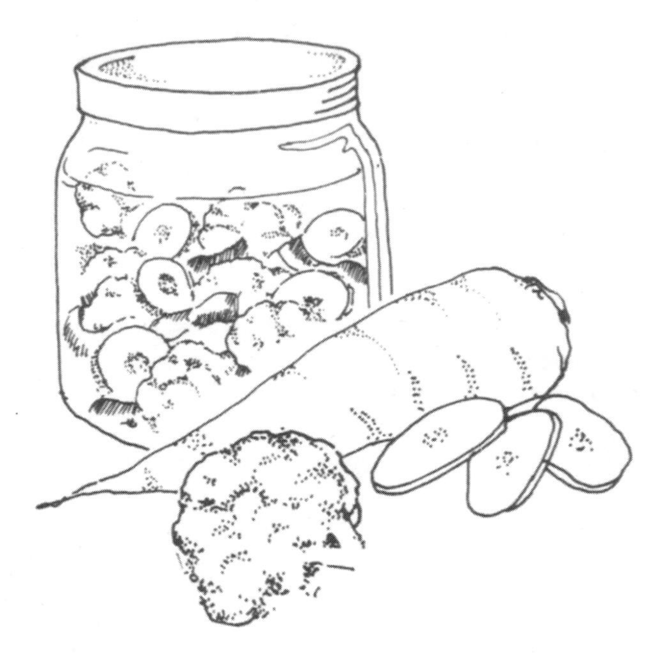

Chestnut Almond Balls

Serves 2-3

Imperial (Metric)	American
7 oz dried chestnuts	1 cup dried chestnuts
1¼ pints (700ml) water	3 cups water
1 5-inch strip of kombu	1 5-inch strip of kombu
Pinch of sea salt	Pinch of sea salt
2 oz (55g) roasted almonds, chopped	½ cup roasted almonds, chopped

1. Soak the chestnuts for 2 hours in the water.
2. Pressure cook in the same water for 35 minutes with the kombu.
3. Remove from heat, season with the sea salt and cook for a further 10 minutes. If excess liquid remains, cook uncovered over a medium heat for a few minutes until reduced.
4. Mash the chestnuts together with any remaining pieces of kombu into a purée.
5. Wet your hands, form small balls with the purée and roll them in the chopped almonds, giving each ball an even coating all around.
6. Arrange attractively on a tray and serve.

Note: When making the balls try keeping one hand wet for forming and the other hand dry for rolling. This may take some practice but it is quicker in the long run. This dish makes a naturally sweet and sustaining party food or dessert.

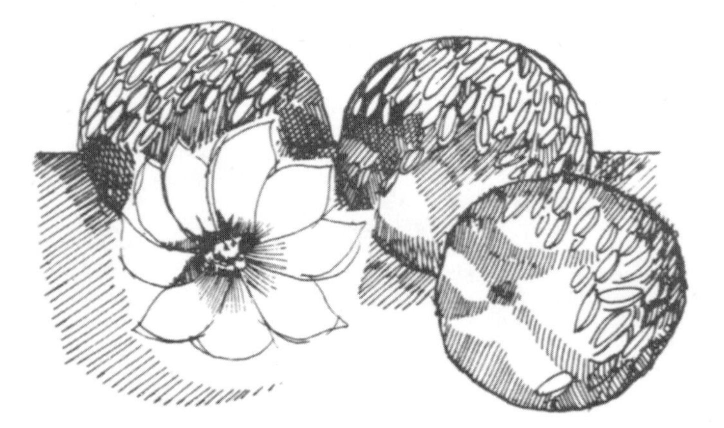

Instant (Tororo) Kombu Soup

Serves 3-4

Imperial (Metric)	American
1½ pints (850ml) water	3¾ cups water
6 oz (170g) tofu, cut into small squares	1 cup tofu, cut into small squares
1 tablespoon shoyu	1 tablespoon shoyu
1 oz (30g) instant (tororo) kombu	1 cup instant (tororo) kombu
1 bunch watercress, cut into 2-inch (5cm) lengths	1 bunch watercress, cut into 2-inch lengths

1. Bring the water to a boil. Add the tofu, shoyu and instant (tororo) kombu and simmer for 5 minutes.
2. Add the watercress and simmer for a further 2-3 minutes. Serve.

Note: This is a very quick to prepare and delicious soup.

Kombu Chips

Imperial (Metric)	American
2-3 short strips of kombu	2-3 short strips of kombu
Vegetable oil for deep frying (preferably unrefined sesame oil)	Vegetable oil for deep frying (preferably unrefined sesame oil)

1. Clean the kombu gently with a damp cloth. Cut with scissors into 1-inch (2.5cm) pieces.
2. Heat the oil to 350°F/180°C.
3. Drop the kombu pieces into the oil and fry until their colour changes and they become crisp. Remove from the oil, drain on a paper towel and serve.

Note: If desired, sprinkle with red pepper or make a dip sauce from fresh ginger juice, shoyu and water, dipping each piece into the sauce before eating. These chips make a perfect appetizer or snack for parties.

Instant (Tororo) Kombu Pumpkin Seed Condiment

Imperial (Metric)	American
1 oz (30g) instant (tororo) kombu	1 cup instant (tororo) kombu
3 oz (85g) roasted pumpkin in seeds	½ cup roasted pumpkin seeds

1. Place the instant kombu on a baking tray and roast in the oven at 350°F/180°C (Gas Mark 4) for just a few minutes until crisp.
2. Remove and grind into a fine powder in a suribachi.
3. Add the roasted pumpkin seeds and grind until the seeds are almost crushed.
4. Serve sprinkled on cereal grain dishes.

Instant (Tororo) Kombu Lemon Condiment

Imperial (Metric)	American
4 fl oz (115ml) water	½ cup water
1 oz (30g) instant (tororo) kombu	1 cup instant (tororo) kombu
¼ tablespoon shoyu	¼ tablespoon shoyu
½ tablespoon lemon juice	½ tablespoon lemon juice

1. Boil the water and mix in the instant (tororo) kombu to form a thick paste.
2. Add the shoyu and lemon juice.
3. Serve as a small side dish to a meal or as a condiment directly on cereal grains.

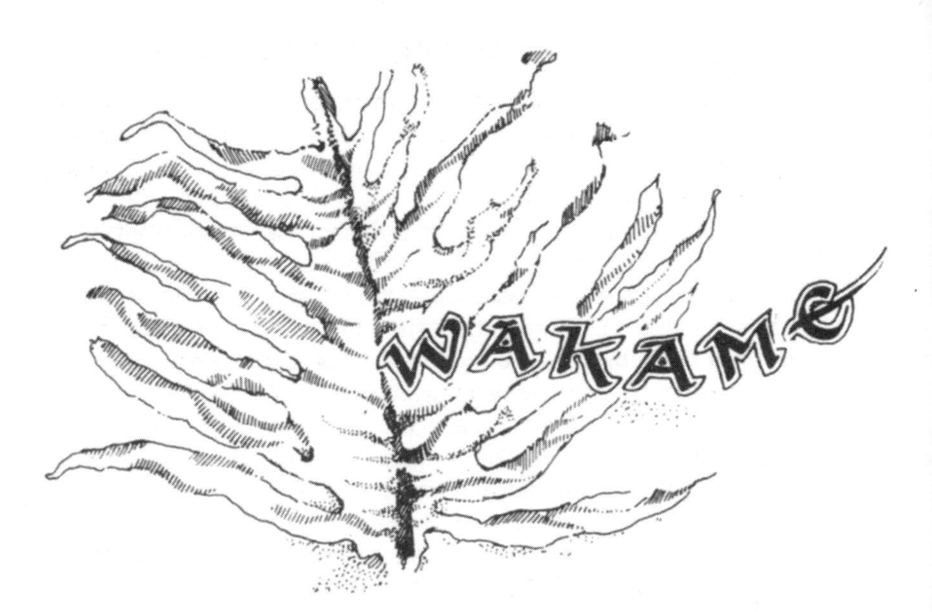

Wakame's mild flavour and leafy form make it one of the most versatile of sea vegetables. It combines well with land vegetables and is especially delicious sautéed with onions, or cooked and served with boiled green vegetables. Simply soaked and served along with cucumber or citrus fruit, with a vinegared dressing, it makes a refreshing summer salad. Lightly baked in an oven and crumbled into a powder, it produces a tasty and mineral-rich condiment for brown rice and cereal dishes. Wakame is also a valuable soup ingredient, and the classic Japanese miso soup is never complete without the addition of wakame. In Japan wakame is the third most popular sea vegetable following closely behind nori and kombu. In the west its light taste makes it one of the most popular with new-comers.

Wakame is classified as a brown sea vegetable and is a close relative of kombu. In dried form the two can easily be confused, although when soaked they are markedly different. Kombu will remain as a thick brown strip, whilst wakame will unfurl into a delicate green leaf attached to a firmer midriff section. The amount of midriff present is one of the distinguishing marks between a higher grade 'leaf' wakame and a lower grade 'stem' wakame. For preparing a delicate dish, any midriff present can be removed by carefully cutting out after soaking.

Wakame is a native of Japanese waters although a similar plant, alaria, commonly known as *wing kelp, dabberlocks* or *murlins*, is widely available from Atlantic waters. Alaria can be substituted for wakame in recipes although it may need a little more cooking. Like kombu, wakame thrives in quick moving currents with, surprisingly, the most tender fronds coming from the most turbulent waters. The plants will grow up to twenty inches (50cm) long in waters twenty to forty feet (6-12m) deep. Growth is most rapid during the winter months and harvesting takes place throughout the spring. This is usually carried out from boats by means of a long-handled rake or hook attached to a rope that by a simple twisting action lifts the holdfast from its rocky base. On the shore the plants are either simply dried and baled or are briefly plunged in boiling water, then immediately dipped in fresh cold water before hanging over a rope to dry. This 'blanching' achieves two things. It turns the wakame an appetizing green (the colour is lost in drying but returns on soaking) and at the same time inhibits the growth of any fermenting micro-organisms, enabling the plant to be sold for a longer time as a fresh vegetable. During the harvesting season in Japan fresh blanched wakame is sold in the markets along with fresh land vegetables. For export, wakame is usually only available in dried form.

Nutritionally, wakame has many of the benefits of its close cousin, kombu. It is especially rich in calcium and contains high levels of the B group of vitamins and also vitamin C. Like kombu it has the ability to soften the fibres of other foods cooked with it.

Ita wakame is tender fronds of carefully selected wakame that have been cut and dried into a sheet form much like nori. It can be toasted and used as a wrapping for rice balls or toasted and crumbled for using as a tasty condiment.

Mekabu is the sporophylls, or reproductive part at the base of the wakame plant, that is prized for its mineral-rich qualities. Its strong salty flavour and sticky texture can add a wonderful richness to root vegetable stews. When cooked in liquid or deep fried, mekabu opens out into a beautiful flower-like shape.

Miso Soup

Serves 2-3

Imperial (Metric)	American
1 oz (30g) wakame	½ cup wakame
1½ pints (850ml) water	3¾ cups water
1 small onion, sliced into half moons	1 small onion, sliced into half moons
2 oz (55g) broccoli, cut into small florets	½ cup broccoli, cut into small florets
1½ teaspoons barley (mugi) miso	1½ teaspoons barley (mugi) miso
Spring onions, chopped to garnish	Scallions, chopped to garnish

1. Wash the wakame quickly under cold water and soak in a very small amount of water for 3 minutes. Slice into small pieces.
2. Bring the water to the boil, add the onions and simmer uncovered for 5-7 minutes.
3. Add the wakame with its soaking water and broccoli and simmer for a further 5 minutes.
4. Purée the miso with a little of the soup liquid in a suribachi or mortar and pestle, then add to the soup. Reduce the heat to very low and simmer for 2 more minutes.
5. Serve, garnishing each bowl of soup with the chopped spring onions (scallions).

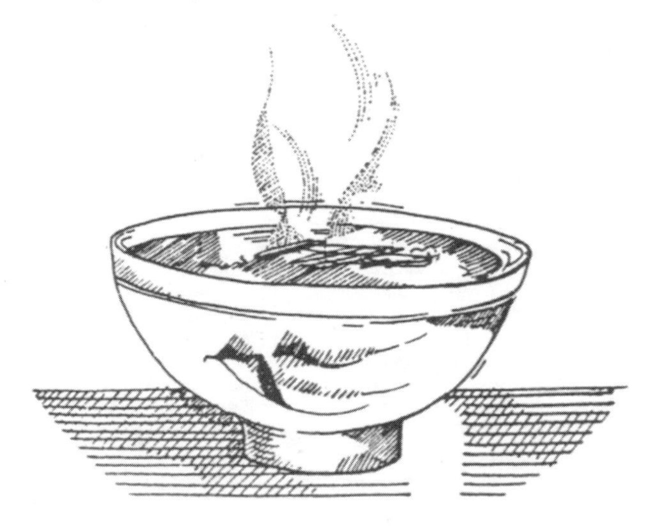

Split Pea Soup

Serves 3-4

Imperial (Metric)	American
½ lb (225g) split peas	1 cup split peas
2½ pints (1.4 litres) water	6 cups water
1 oz (30g) wakame, soaked 3 minutes and sliced into small pieces	½ cup wakame, soaked 3 minutes and sliced into small pieces
1 medium onion, diced	1 medium onion, diced
¼ teaspoon sea salt	¼ teaspoon sea salt
Wholemeal bread, cut into small cubes and baked, to garnish	Wholewheat bread, cut into small cubes and baked, to garnish

1. Wash the split peas and put in a heavy pot with the water and the wakame.
2. Bring to the boil, reduce the heat to low, cover, and simmer for 1 hour. (Check regularly to ensure the peas do not stick to the bottom.)
3. Add the diced onions and simmer uncovered for 5 minutes.
4. Add the sea salt and simmer for a further 10-15 minutes.
5. Serve garnished with the baked bread croûtons.

Note: A small quantity of grated carrot or chopped spring onions (scallions) can also be used to garnish.

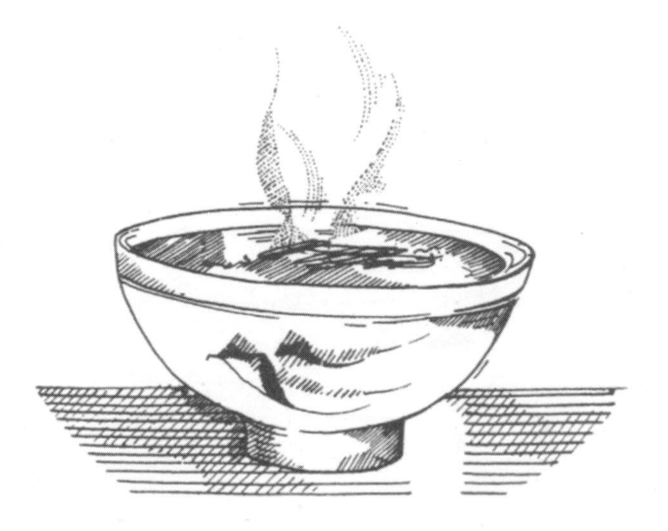

Brown Rice Salad

Serves 3-4

Imperial (Metric)	American
½ lb (225g) cooked brown rice	1½ cups cooked brown rice
Pinch of sea salt	Pinch of sea salt
3 oz (85g) carrots, diced	½ cup carrots, diced
1 oz (30g) celery, diced	¼ cup celery, diced
3 oz (85g) red radish, sliced into thin rounds	½ cup red radish, sliced into thin rounds
1 oz (30g) wakame, soaked for 3 minutes and sliced into small pieces	½ cup wakame, soaked for 3 minutes and sliced into small pieces
½ oz (15g) parsley, chopped	½ cup parsley, chopped
4 oz (115g) roasted peanuts, roughly chopped	¼ cup roasted peanuts, roughly chopped
3 oz (85g) diced cucumber (mix with pinch of sea salt, leave for 1 hour, squeeze out liquid)	½ cup diced cucumber (mix with pinch of sea salt, leave for 1 hour, squeeze out liquid)
Dressing:	*Dressing:*
4 tablespoons natural mustard	4 tablespoons natural mustard
3 tablespoons umeboshi vinegar	3 tablespoons umeboshi vinegar
3 tablespoons lemon juice	3 tablespoons lemon juice

1. Stir the cooked brown rice to make it fluffy (best done immediately after cooking).
2. To a pot of boiling water add a pinch of sea salt then cook the vegetables separately in the order and for the length of time shown, removing one before adding the next: carrots 2-3 minutes, celery 1-2 minutes, radish ½ minute. After each vegetable has been cooked, spread out on a plate and leave to cool before placing in a serving bowl.
3. Add the cooked rice, wakame, parsley, roasted peanuts and cucumber.
4. Mix the dressing ingredients and carefully stir into the salad.

Note: This makes a refreshing light summer dish.

Watercress with Scrambled Tofu

Serves 2-3

Imperial (Metric)	American
1 oz (30g) wakame	½ cup wakame
Few drops of sesame oil	Few drops of sesame oil
6 oz (170g) tofu, crushed in a suribachi or with a fork	1 cup tofu, crushed in a suribachi or with a fork
3 bunches watercress	3 bunches watercress
1 teaspoon brown rice (genmai) miso	1 teaspoon brown rice (genmai) miso
1½ teaspoons juice freshly grated ginger	1½ teaspoons juice freshly grated ginger
3 tablespoons sesame seeds, roasted (optional)	3 tablespoons sesame seeds, roasted (optional)

1. Wash the wakame quickly under cold water and soak for 3 minutes. Slice into small pieces.
2. Brush a frying pan with a small amount of sesame oil. Heat and add the tofu, stirring gently for 2-3 minutes.
3. Add the watercress and wakame, sautéing for 1-2 minutes.
4. Purée the miso in a small amount of water, add to the frying pan with the ginger juice. Sauté for 1-2 minutes more.
5. Add the roasted sesame seeds if desired.

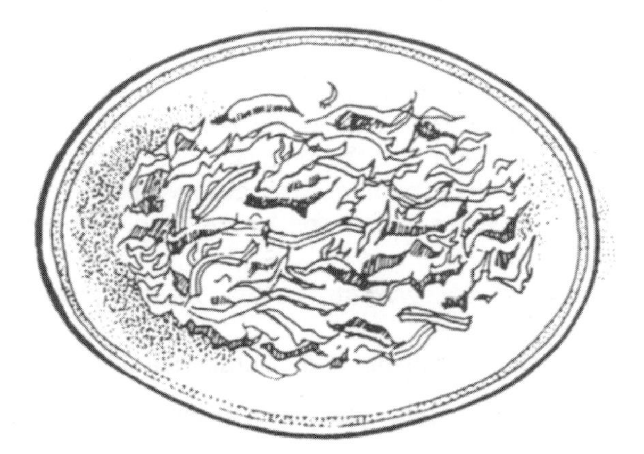

Wakame Vegetable Stew

Serves 4-5

Imperial (Metric)

1 oz (30g) wakame, soaked for 3 minutes and sliced into small pieces
1½ pints (850ml) water
2 medium onions, quartered
2 medium turnips, quartered
½ lb (225g) Brussels sprouts
7 oz (200g) pumpkin, seeds removed and cut into 1 inch × 1½ inch (2.5 × 4cm) chunks
3 tablespoons shoyu
2 tablespoons mirin (optional)

American

½ cup wakame, soaked for 3 minutes and sliced into small pieces
3¾ cups water
2 medium onions, quartered
2 medium turnips, quartered
½ pound Brussels sprouts
4 cups winter squash, seeds removed and cut into 1 inch × 1½ inch chunks
3 tablespoons shoyu
2 tablespoons mirin (optional)

1. Place the wakame in the bottom of a heavy pot. Add the water and bring to the boil.
2. Add the onions and simmer for 3-4 minutes uncovered.
3. Add the turnips, Brussels sprouts and pumpkin (squash) in layers, seasoning with the shoyu and mirin (optional). Bring to the boil and simmer for 15-20 minutes, covered.
4. Boil off excess liquid over a medium to high heat.

Note: As an alternative to boiling off the excess liquid, it can be thickened into a sauce by dissolving a little kuzu in cold water, then adding it to the vegetables and stirring gently for ½-1 minute until clear. This dish can also be cooked with cubes of tofu or seitan on the top.

Chinese Style Sautéed Vegetables

Serves 3-4

Imperial (Metric)	American
Few drops of sesame oil	Few drops of sesame oil
4 oz (115g) leeks, sliced diagonally	1 cup leeks, sliced diagonally
6 mushrooms, thinly sliced	6 mushrooms, thinly sliced
3 oz (85g) carrots, cut into fine matchsticks	½ cup carrots, cut into fine matchsticks
Pinch of sea salt	Pinch of sea salt
4 oz (115g) Chinese cabbage, sliced diagonally	1 cup Chinese cabbage, sliced diagonally
1 oz (30g) beansprouts	½ cup beansprouts
1 oz (30g) wakame, soaked for 5 minutes and sliced into small pieces	½ cup wakame, soaked for 5 minutes and sliced into small pieces
3 oz (85g) seitan, wheat gluten cut into fine matchsticks	½ cup seitan, wheat meat, cut into fine matchsticks
3 tablespoons shoyu	3 tablespoons shoyu
1½ tablespoons juice from grated ginger root	1½ tablespoons juice from grated ginger root
2 tablespoons kuzu, dissolved in ½ pint (285ml) water	2 tablespoons kuzu, dissolved in 1⅓ cups water

1. Lightly oil a frying pan and heat. Add the leeks and mushrooms and sauté uncovered for 1-2 minutes.
2. Add the carrots and a pinch of sea salt and sauté for 3-4 minutes, covering between stirring.
3. Add the Chinese cabbage, beansprouts, wakame, seitan and shoyu. Sauté for 2-3 minutes, moving the vegetables from side to side to avoid burning and ensure even cooking.
4. Add the ginger juice and diluted kuzu, reduce the heat to low and stir gently for ½-1 minute.

Note: This dish can either be served alone or with noodles.

Stuffed Turnips

Serves 2

Imperial (Metric)	American
4 medium turnips	4 medium turnips
Pinch of sea salt	Pinch of sea salt
Few drops of sesame oil	Few drops of sesame oil
2 onions, cut into half moons	2 onions, cut into half moons
1 oz (30g) wakame, soaked for 3 minutes and sliced into small pieces	½ cup wakame, soaked for 3 minutes and sliced into small pieces
1½ tablespoons shoyu	1½ tablespoons shoyu
2 tablespoons lemon rind	2 tablespoons lemon rind
1 oz (30g) almonds, roasted and chopped	¼ cup almonds, roasted and chopped
Parsley, finely chopped to garnish	Parsley, finely chopped to garnish

1. Carefully slice the top ½ inch (1cm) off the turnips. Remove the inside of the turnips with a spoon. (Keep the insides for use in another dish.)
2. Place the turnips and the top pieces in boiling water with a pinch of sea salt. Remove the top pieces after 3-4 minutes and the turnips after 6-7 minutes. Leave both on plate to cool.
3. Lightly oil a frying pan and heat. Add the onions and sauté for about 5 minutes until translucent.
4. Add the wakame and shoyu. Sauté for a further 2 minutes.
5. Add the lemon rind and chopped almonds. Briefly stir and remove from heat.
6. Stuff each turnip with the cooked mixture and replace the top pieces.
7. Garnish each turnip with chopped parsley and serve.

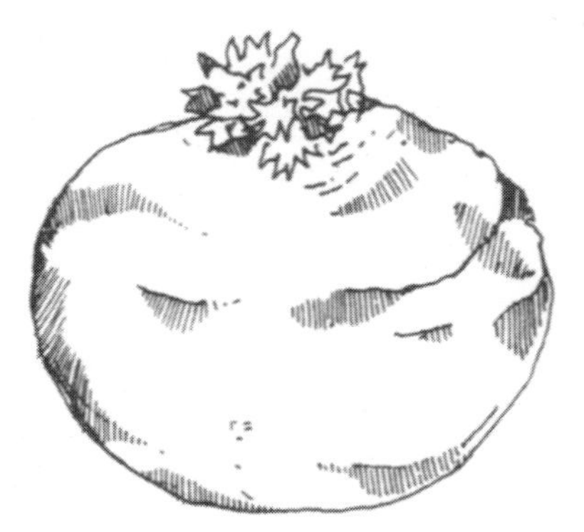

Vinegared Land and Sea Vegetables

Serves 2-3

Imperial (Metric)	American
Pinch of sea salt	Pinch of sea salt
3 oz (85g) carrots, cut into thin rounds	½ cup carrots, cut into thin rounds
3 oz (85g) cauliflower, cut into florets	½ cup cauliflower, cut into florets
2 oz (55g) mangetout or French beans (remove strings that run along spine of each pod)	½ cup snow peas or snap beans (remove strings that run along spine of each pod)
1 oz (30g) beansprouts	½ cup beansprouts
1 oz (30g) wakame (soaked for 3-5 minutes, cut into small pieces)	½ cup wakame (soaked for 3-5 minutes, cut into small pieces)
Dressing:	*Dressing:*
4 tablespoons brown rice vinegar	4 tablespoons brown rice vinegar
1 tablespoon shoyu	1 tablespoon shoyu
1 tablespoon water	1 tablespoon water

1. **Bring one pot of water to the boil and add a pinch of sea salt.**
2. **Boil each vegetable in turn (removing one before adding the next) in the following order for these lengths of time: carrots 2-3 minutes, cauliflower 2-3 minutes, peas (or beans) 1-2 minutes.**
3. **After each vegetable has been boiled, spread out on a plate and leave to cool.**
4. **Place all the vegetables and the soaked wakame mixed together in a serving bowl.**
5. **Mix the dressing ingredients together and pour over the vegetables before serving.**

Pressed Salad with Wakame

(See front cover photograph)
Serves 2-3

Imperial (Metric)	American
1 cucumber, sliced into thin rounds	1 cucumber, sliced into thin rounds
2 medium carrots, cut into very fine matchsticks	2 medium carrots, cut into very fine matchsticks
1 teaspoon sea salt	1 teaspoon sea salt
1 oz (30g) wakame, soaked for 3 minutes and sliced into small pieces	½ cup wakame, soaked for 3 minutes and sliced into small pieces
Slice of orange or lemon, to garnish	Slice of orange or lemon, to garnish
Dressing:	*Dressing:*
4 tablespoons orange or lemon juice	4 tablespoons orange or lemon juice

1. Place the cucumber and carrots in a pickle press or large bowl and sprinkle with the salt. Mix well and apply pressure to the press or if using a bowl, put a plate on top of the vegetables and then a heavy weight. Leave for 1-2 hours.
2. Pour off the excess liquid from both the cucumber and the carrots and leave them briefly to drain.
3. In a serving bowl separately place the cucumber, carrots and wakame in an attractive display. Pour the dressing over the top and decorate the dish with a half moon slice of orange or lemon.

Roasted Wakame Condiment

Imperial (Metric)	American
¾ oz (25g) wakame	½ cup wakame
2 oz (55g) pumpkin seeds	¼ cup pumpkin seeds

1. Heat oven to 375°F/190°C (Gas Mark 5) and roast the wakame on a tray until crisp.
2. Grind into a fine powder in a suribachi or with a mortar and pestle.
3. Wash the pumpkin seeds and dry roast in a frying pan on a low heat until they release a nutty fragrance, stirring constantly to ensure even cooking.
4. Add the pumpkin seeds to the wakame and grind together until the seeds are semi-crushed.
5. Serve as a condiment with brown rice and cereal dishes.

Mekabu Kidney Bean Soup

Serves 3-5

Imperial (Metric)	American
3 oz (85g) red kidney beans	½ cup red kidney beans
1 oz (30g) mekabu	½ cup mekabu
2½ pints (1.4 litres) water	6 cups water
6 oz (170g) carrots, pumpkin or parsnips; diced	1 cup carrots, winter squash or parsnips, diced
6 oz (170g) onions, diced	1 cup onions, diced
½ tablespoon shoyu	½ tablespoon shoyu
Spring onions, chopped to garnish	Scallions, chopped to garnish

1. Soak the kidney beans overnight in half of the water.
2. Soak the mekabu in the other half of the water for 10-15 minutes. Remove and cut into small pieces.
3. To a large pot add the mekabu and its soaking water and the kidney beans and their soaking water. Bring to the boil and simmer for 1¼ hours or until the beans are soft.
4. Add the carrots (or other chosen vegetable) and onions and simmer uncovered for 5 minutes.
5. Add more water if necessary, then add the shoyu and simmer gently for a further 10 minutes.
6. Serve garnished with the chopped spring onions (scallions).

Mekabu Stew

Serves 3-4

Imperial (Metric)
1 oz (30g) mekabu
1½ pints (850ml) water
6 oz (170g) swede, cubed
5 small whole onions
6 oz (170g) daikon radish, cut in half rounds ½ inch (1cm) thick
½ teaspoon shoyu
2 tablespoons juice from freshly squeezed grated ginger
Parsley, chopped fine to garnish

American
½ cup mekabu
3¾ cups water
1 cup rutabaga, cubed
5 small whole onions
1 cup daikon radish, cut in half rounds ½ inch thick
½ teaspoon shoyu
2 tablespoons juice from freshly squeezed grated ginger
Parsley, chopped fine to garnish

1. Soak the mekabu in half the amount of water for about 1 hour until soft. Remove and cut into small pieces. Retain the soaking water.
2. Place half the soaking water, the rest of the water and the mekabu in a large pan. Bring to the boil and simmer for 20 minutes.
3. Add the vegetables in layers and the shoyu and cook for 10-15 minutes. If necessary add more water during cooking. Add the ginger juice and cook for a few more minutes until the liquid has evaporated.
4. Serve in a bowl garnished with the chopped parsley.

Note: This recipe can be made with other combinations of seasonal root vegetables.

Mekabu Chips

Imperial (Metric)	American
2 oz (50g) packet of mekabu	1 cup mekabu
Sesame oil for deep frying	Sesame oil for deep frying
1 lemon, sliced into half moons ½ inch (1cm) thick	1 lemon, sliced into half moons ½ inch thick

1. Clean the mekabu with a damp cloth to remove any white salt deposits.
2. Heat the sesame oil to 350°F/180°C. Drop the mekabu in the oil and deep fry for a few minutes until it becomes crisp. Remove from the oil and drain on a paper towel.
3. Place on a serving tray with the lemon slices, and eat after first squeezing lemon juice on each piece.

Note: Mekabu will open up into a flower-like shape on deep frying. If the pieces are too large for serving, carefully cut them smaller. This dish has an attractive salty taste and is a popular party food.

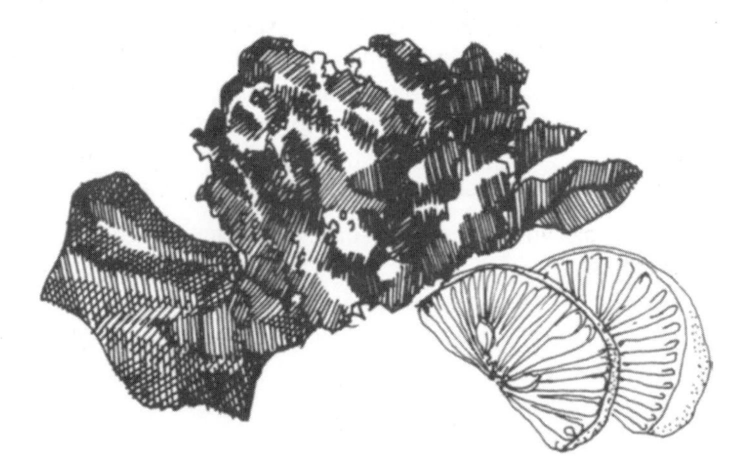

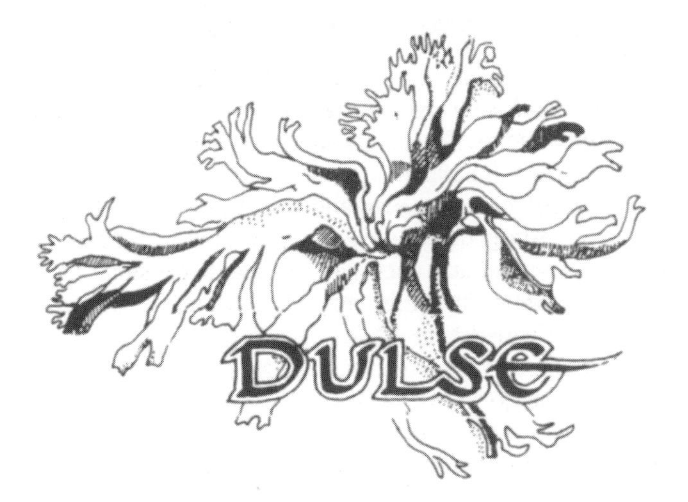

Purple red dulse has a soft texture with a uniquely spicy flavour. It can be used to prepare a delightful range of soups and condiments and lightly cooked it combines well with onions and is a tasty accompaniment to oats and other cooked grains. Simply soaked it makes a colourful and nutritious addition to a variety of salads.

Dulse is the most popular native sea vegetable of the North Atlantic and has been used for well over a thousand years as a food by the peoples of north west Europe. It is said that ancient Celtic and Nordic warriors chewed dulse on their marches and that the monks of St Columba gathered it to feed to the poor. Icelandic and Alaskan peoples have also for many centuries regularly included dulse in their diet. In the seventeenth century it was used by British sailors as a chewing tobacco and it was observed at the time that dulse was a contributing factor to the lower incidence of scurvy found in British seafarers compared with those of other nationalities. In the eighteenth century Scottish and Irish immigrants established dulse's popularity along the eastern seaboard of Canada and New England and until the late nineteenth century dulse was commonly traded in the streets of seaports on both sides of the Atlantic. As with most sea vegetables in the West, however, its use has declined this century although recently with an increased public awareness in natural foods, local harvesting industries are once again back in business.

Dulse grows profusely around the low water line in the turbulent waters on rocky shores. The plants are small, measuring between six and twelve inches (15-30cm) long and have flat, smooth fronds. Harvesting occurs between May and October when the plants are picked by hand during the low tide. They are simply dried by the sun and wind then sorted and packaged for sale. Because of its natural habitat around the tide line, dulse may contain small shells and should be thoroughly cleaned before use.

Dulse is the richest of all the sea vegetables in iron, which makes it an important blood strengthener. It also contains an abundance of potassium, magnesium, iodine and phosphorus. After nori, dulse has the highest protein content of any common sea vegetable.

Dulse Oatmeal Soup

Serves 3-4

Imperial (Metric)	American
2 pints (1.1 litres) water	5 cups water
½ medium onion, sliced in half moons	½ medium onion, sliced in half moons
4 oz (115g) rolled oats	1 cup rolled oats
1½ oz (45g) dulse, soaked in ⅓ pint (200ml) water for 5 minutes and finely sliced	½ cup dulse, soaked in ¾ cup water for 5 minutes and finely sliced
Pinch of sea salt	Pinch of sea salt
Parsley, spring onions or watercress chopped fine to garnish	Parsley, scallions or watercress chopped fine to garnish

1. Bring the water to the boil, add the onions and simmer uncovered for 5 minutes.
2. Add the rolled oats, dulse, soaking water from the dulse and the sea salt. Bring to the boil, reduce the flame and simmer for 20-25 minutes.
3. Garnish with chopped parsley, spring onions (scallions) or watercress. Grated carrot can also be used as a garnish, if desired.

Oatmeal Dulse Croquettes

Serves 2-4

Imperial (Metric)	American
2 oz (55g) rolled oats	½ cup rolled oats
6 oz (170g) onions, diced	1 cup onions, diced
1½ oz (45g) dulse, soaked for 5 minutes in water and finely sliced	½ cup dulse, soaked for 5 minutes in water and finely sliced
2 tablespoons wholemeal flour	2 tablespoons wholewheat flour
Pinch of sea salt	Pinch of sea salt
Sesame oil for deep frying	Sesame oil for deep frying

1. **Mix the rolled oats, onions, dulse, flour and sea salt with enough of the dulse soaking water to form a stiff mix.**
2. **Shape into 2 inch (5cm) diameter flat croquettes with your hands, adding more dulse soaking water or flour, if necessary, to obtain a firm consistency.**
3. **Heat enough oil to thoroughly cover the croquettes to 375°F/190°C. Deep fry the croquettes until a golden brown all over. (As they are best eaten fresh, do not cook too many at once.)**
4. **Drain on a paper towel. Serve on a dish with a paper napkin underneath to soak up any remaining oil.**

Note: **Serve with a dipping sauce of either fresh ginger juice, shoyu and water or grated daikon radish with a few drops of shoyu.**

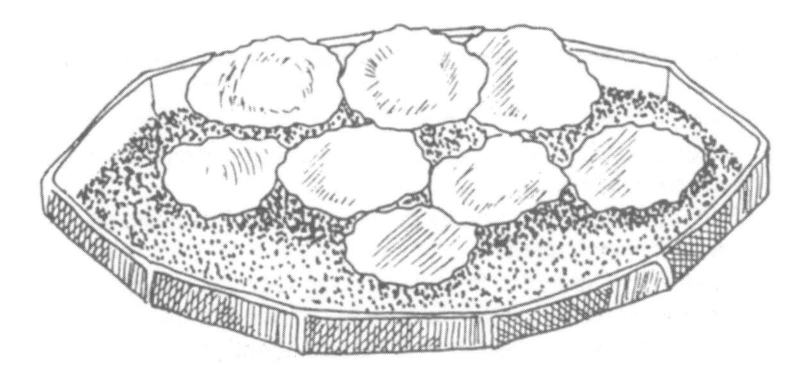

Noodle Salad

Serves 3-4

Imperial (Metric)	American
5 oz (140g) cucumber, cut into fine rounds	½ cup cucumber, cut into fine rounds
6 oz (170g) red radish, cut into fine rounds	½ cup red radish, cut into fine rounds
Pinch of sea salt	Pinch of sea salt
4 oz (115g) udon or wholewheat spaghetti	4 ounces udon or wholewheat spaghetti
1½ oz (45g) dulse, soaked in water for 5 minutes, then finely sliced	½ cup dulse, soaked in water for 5 minutes, then finely sliced
4 oz (115g) tofu, cut into small cubes and boiled for 1-2 minutes	½ cup tofu, cut into small cubes and boiled for 1-2 minutes
Dressing:	*Dressing:*
2 tablespoons sesame spread	2 tablespoons sesame butter
2 fl oz (60ml) brown rice vinegar	¼ cup brown rice vinegar
2 tablespoons shoyu	2 tablespoons shoyu
4 fl oz (115ml) water	½ cup water

1. Place the cucumber and red radish in a pickle press or bowl with the sea salt. Mix well, apply pressure to the press or place a weight on a saucer on the vegetables and leave for 1 hour.
2. Meanwhile, place the spaghetti in boiling water, return to the boil, reduce the heat and cook. To test if done, remove one spaghetti strand and break it in half. The centre should be the same colour as the outside. If you are using wholewheat spaghetti the boiling water should be lightly salted. This is not necessary for udon, which already contains salt.
3. Place the noodles in a strainer and rinse under cold water to prevent them sticking together.
4. Squeeze the liquid out from the pressed vegetables, discard, and mix the vegetables with the noodles, dulse and tofu.
5. Mix the dressing ingredients together and gently toss in with the salad.

Dulse Cocktail

See front cover photograph
Serves 2-3

Imperial (Metric)
2 cobs fresh sweetcorn
Pinch of sea salt
½ lettuce, shredded
3 oz (85g) cucumber, sliced diagonally finely, mixed with a pinch of sea salt left 20 minutes, liquid squeezed out
1½ oz (45g) dulse, soaked for 5 minutes and finely sliced

Dressing:
1 tablespoon umeboshi vinegar
4 tablespoons natural mustard
5 tablespoons water

Decoration (optional):
1 tablespoon parsley, chopped
Lemon, sliced in half moons

American
2 ears fresh sweetcorn
Pinch of sea salt
½ lettuce, shredded
⅓ cup cucumber, sliced diagonally finely, mixed with a pinch of sea salt left 20 minutes, liquid squeezed out
1½ cups dulse, soaked for 5 minutes and finely sliced

Dressing:
1 tablespoon umeboshi vinegar
4 tablespoons natural mustard
5 tablespoons water

Decoration (optional):
1 tablespoon parsley, chopped
Lemon, sliced in half moons

1. Place the sweetcorn in boiling water with a pinch of sea salt and cook for 15-20 minutes until soft. Remove the corn kernels from the cobs.
2. Place the lettuce evenly in the bottom of a flat serving bowl.
3. Neatly arrange the cucumber slices in a circle around the edge.
4. Mix the dressing ingredients together.
5. Mix the dulse and corn together with the dressing. Place in the centre of the serving bowl on top of the lettuce.
6. Decorate with the parsley and lemon (optional).

Variation: Small dices of carrot, boiled for 1-2 minutes, can be used instead of the corn.

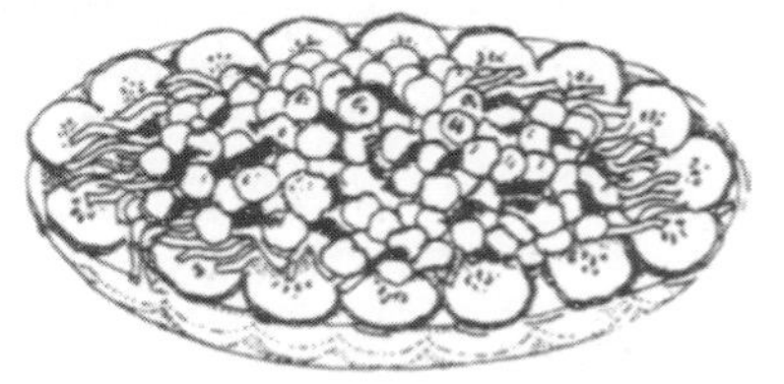

Glazed Cauliflower and Radish

Serves 2-3

Imperial (Metric)
- 3 tablespoons shiso leaves from the top of an umeboshi container
- ⅔ pint (340ml) water
- 5 oz (140g) cauliflower, cut into florets
- 1 bunch small red radishes, kept whole
- 1½ oz (45g) dulse, soaked for 5 minutes and finely sliced
- 2 tablespoons kuzu, dissolved in 4 tablespoons cold water

American
- 3 tablespoons shiso leaves from the top of an umeboshi container
- 1½ cups water
- 1 cup cauliflower, cut into florets
- 1 bunch small red radishes, kept whole
- ½ cup dulse, soaked for 5 minutes and finely sliced
- 2 tablespoons kuzu, dissolved in 4 tablespoons cold water

1. Add the shiso leaves to boiling water and simmer for 20 minutes. Remove the leaves and keep for another dish.
2. In the same boiling water, cook the cauliflower for 4-5 minutes. Remove.
3. Cook the red radishes for 1 minute in the same water and then remove.
4. Cook the dulse in the same water for ½ minute.
5. Place the cauliflower, red radish and dulse neatly in a serving bowl.
6. Add the kuzu liquid to the cooking water and stir on a low heat until clear and thick. Pour over the vegetables.

Note: This dish can be garnished with chopped parsley and either served on its own or with noodles.

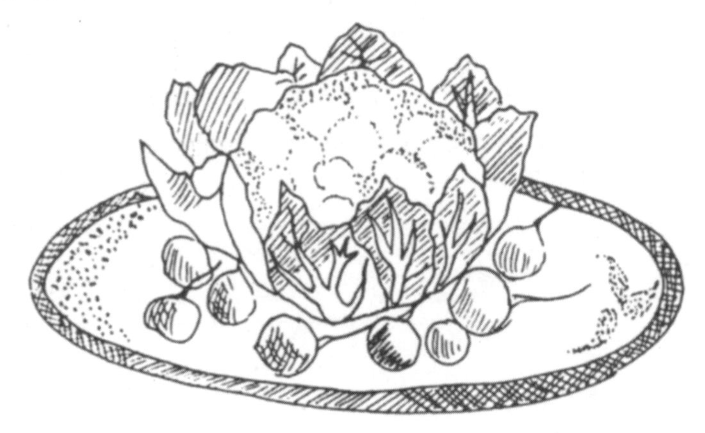

Fresh Corn Salad

Serves 3-4

Imperial (Metric)
4 cobs fresh sweetcorn
Pinch of sea salt
3 oz (85g) carrots, cut in thin rounds
4 oz (115g) broccoli, cut in small florets
3 oz (85g) dulse, soaked for 5 minutes and finely sliced

Dressing:
3 tablespoons grated onion
1 tablespoon shoyu
4 fl oz (115ml) pickle juice or brown rice vinegar and water (2 parts vinegar to 1 part water)

American
4 ears fresh sweetcorn
Pinch of sea salt
½ cup carrots, cut in thin rounds
1 cup broccoli, cut in small florets
1 cup dulse, soaked for 5 minutes and finely sliced

Dressing:
3 tablespoons grated onion
1 tablespoon shoyu
½ cup pickle juice or brown rice vinegar and water (2 parts vinegar to 1 part water)

1. Place the sweetcorn in boiling water, add a pinch of salt and cook for 20 minutes or until soft. Retain the boiling water.
2. Remove the corn kernels from the cobs.
3. Cook the carrots for 3-4 minutes in the same boiling water. Take out and spread out on a plate to cool. Cook and cool the broccoli the same way.
4. Mix the corn, carrots, broccoli and dulse in a serving bowl.
5. Mix the dressing ingredients together and pour over the salad before serving.

Beansprout Salad with Dulse

Serves 3-4

Imperial (Metric)	American
5 oz (140g) beansprouts	2½ cups beansprouts
Pinch of sea salt	Pinch of sea salt
4 oz (115g) grated carrots	1 cup grated carrots
3 oz (85g) dulse, soaked for 5 minutes and finely sliced	1 cup dulse, soaked for 5 minutes and finely sliced
1 oz (30g) walnuts, roasted and chopped	3 tablespoons walnuts, roasted and chopped
1 bunch watercress, chopped finely	1 bunch watercress, chopped finely
Dressing:	*Dressing:*
⅓ pint (200ml) tangerine juice	¾ cup tangerine juice
2 tablespoons shoyu	2 tablespoons shoyu

1. **Place the beansprouts in boiling water with a pinch of sea salt for 1-2 minutes. Remove and cool on a plate.**
2. **Mix the beansprouts, grated carrot, dulse, walnuts and watercress and place in a serving bowl.**
3. **Mix the dressing ingredients and pour over the salad before serving.**

Dulse Dressing

Imperial (Metric)	American
4 fl oz (115ml) water	½ cup water
2 tablespoons sesame spread	2 tablespoons sesame butter
1 tablespoon umeboshi paste	1 tablespoon umeboshi paste
1½ oz (45g) dulse, soaked for 5 minutes in water and finely sliced	½ cup dulse, soaked for 5 minutes in water and finely sliced
3 spring onions, finely chopped	3 scallions, finely chopped

1. **Heat the water, add the sesame spread (sesame butter) and blend together. Put in a suribachi.**
2. **Add the umeboshi paste to the suribachi and blend in.**
3. **Add the dulse and spring onions (scallions) and mix in.**

Note: **The soaking water from the dulse can be used instead of plain water in this dressing. Also, if the dressing is too salty, then use less**

umeboshi paste. Parsley or watercress can be used as an alternative to spring onions (scallions). This is a very appealing dressing for salads.

Stuffed Chinese Cabbage Rolls

Makes 8 rolls, serves 2-4

Imperial (Metric)	American
4 large Chinese cabbage leaves	4 large Chinese cabbage leaves
Pinch of sea salt	Pinch of sea salt
1½ oz (45g) dulse, soaked for 5 minutes in water and finely sliced	½ cup dulse, soaked for 5 minutes in water and finely sliced
3 oz (85g) natural sauerkraut	½ cup natural sauerkraut

1. Blanch the Chinese cabbage leaves for ½ minute in boiling water with a pinch of sea salt. Remove and spread out on a tray to cool. Drain.
2. Mix the dulse and sauerkraut together.
3. Lay one cabbage leaf at a time on a cutting board and place a quarter of the dulse and sauerkraut mix evenly across each leaf.
4. Roll up the cabbage leaf around the mixture into a tight roll. Cut each roll in half crosswise and stand vertically.
5. Decorate the top of each roll with a small quantity of sauerkraut.

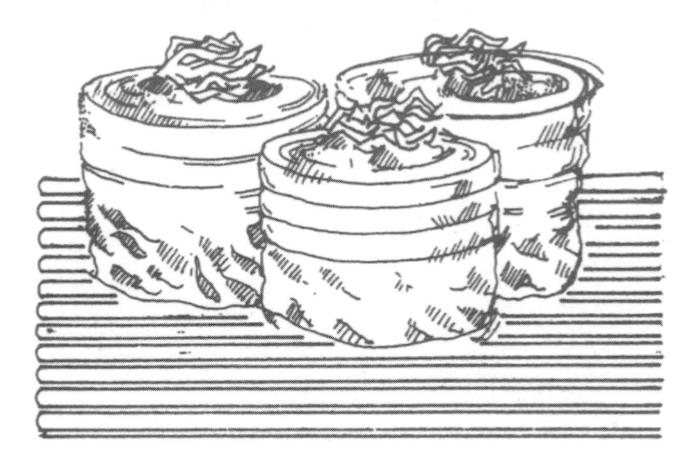

Dulse Condiment

Imperial (Metric)	American
Few drops of sesame oil	Few drops of sesame oil
1 medium onion, diced	1 medium onion, diced
½ oz (15g) parsley, chopped	½ cup parsley, chopped
1½ oz (45g) dulse, soaked for 5 minutes and finely chopped	½ cup dulse, soaked for 5 minutes and finely chopped
½ tablespoon brown rice (genmai) miso, diluted in 3 tablespoons dulse soaking water	½ tablespoon brown rice (genmai) miso, diluted in 3 tablespoons dulse soaking water
1 tablespoon juice from freshly grated and squeezed ginger root	1 tablespoon juice from freshly grated and squeezed ginger root

1. Lightly oil a frying pan and heat. Add the diced onions and parsley and sauté for 5 minutes until translucent.
2. Add the dulse and sauté for 1-2 minutes, then season with the diluted miso and ginger juice. Simmer until all the liquid has evaporated.
3. Serve on cereal grains or as a small side dish.

Note: A roasted dulse condiment can be made by roasting dulse in an oven at 375°F/190°C (Gas Mark 5) for 5-7 minutes until crisp and then grinding into a fine powder in a suribachi. This can be served like roasted kombu and wakame condiments, sprinkled on cereal grains.

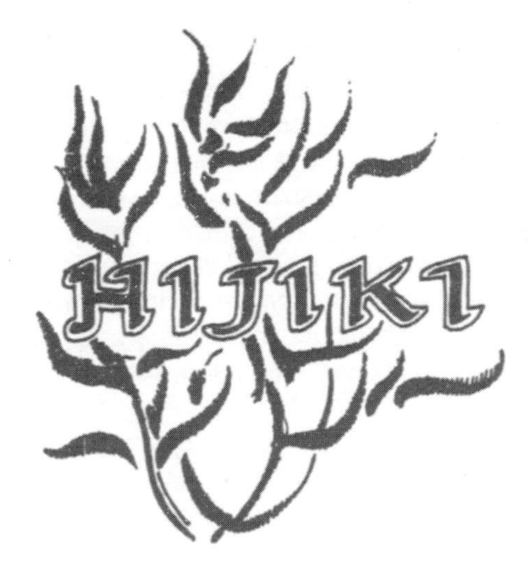

The black cylindrical strings of hijiki have long been treasured as one of nature's richest sources of minerals. They may taste a little strong at first but acquiring a taste is well worth the effort. One hundred grams dry weight of hijiki contains over one thousand four hundred milligrams of calcium compared with milk which has only one hundred milligrams per hundred grams. As well as containing quantities of most of the major minerals, hijiki has an abundance of trace elements and their overall effect is to tone up the system and purify the blood sugar level. Hijiki has always been regularly eaten in small amounts in Japan where it has become legendary for enhancing beauty and adding lustre and resilience to the hair.

Hijiki primarily grows in the Far East where its bush-like plants carpet the rocks just below the water line. Each bush grows to about forty inches high and harvesting takes place between January and May when the annual growth is at its peak. Generally the most tender and best tasting shoots are those that grow first and they are picked early in the season during January and February. After harvesting the brown shoots are dried in the sun and then boiled in large vats of fresh water for several hours to make them more tender. During boiling they become black by reabsorbing the concentrated pigment released into the boiling water. After cooking they are once again dried and then graded and packaged for sale.

Hijiki will expand considerably on soaking, yielding up to five times its dry volume, so be careful not to start out with too much. Hijiki harmonizes well with oil and is usually sautéed. It requires longer cooking than most sea vegetables. Hijiki is sweetened considerably when cooked with onions and also combines well with root vegetables. Note that the best method of washing and soaking hijiki is to place it in a bowl, cover with water and stir. Then remove the hijiki to a second bowl and repeat with fresh water. Repeat again, this time using a cooking pot and the correct amount of water for soaking, as stated in the recipe. Leave to soak for 10 minutes. As with other sea vegetables the water from soaking can be used in cooking, but if it is too salty, dilute by adding some fresh water.

Hijiki Onion Rolls

Imperial (Metric)

Crêpes:

4 oz (115g) wholemeal pastry flour
1 tablespoon arrowroot
Pinch of sea salt
⅔ pint (340ml) sparkling water or beer
Few drops of sesame oil

Filling:

1¾ oz (50g) hijiki
Water to cover hijiki
Few drops sesame oil
3 medium onions, sliced in half moons
1¼ tablespoons shoyu
Spring onions, chopped to garnish

American

Crêpes:

1 cup wholewheat pastry flour
1 tablespoon arrowroot
Pinch of sea salt
1½ cups sparkling water or beer
Few drops of sesame oil

Filling:

½ cup hijiki
Water to cover hijiki
Few drops sesame oil
3 medium onions, sliced in half moons
1¼ tablespoons shoyu
Scallions, chopped to garnish

1. To prepare the crêpes, in a bowl mix the flour, arrowroot, a pinch of sea salt and the water or beer, using enough liquid to make a very thin batter. Set aside for 30 minutes.
2. Brush a flat frying pan or crêpe pan with a few drops of the sesame oil, heat, and pour in a little of the crêpe batter,

smoothing with a spoon or tilting the pan to ensure an even thin round coating. Cook one side, turn and cook the other. Remove from the pan and keep on a plate covered with a clean tea towel.

3. To prepare the filling, wash and soak the hijiki (see page 100). Remove (keeping the soaking water) and slice into 1 inch (2.5cm) lengths.
4. Lightly brush a frying pan with a few drops of sesame oil, heat, add the sliced onions and sauté for 10 minutes. Add ¼ tablespoon of the shoyu and simmer gently for a few more minutes.
5. Place the hijiki and the soaking water in a pot discarding the last part which may contain small sand particles. (If this water tastes too salty use half only and top up with fresh water to cover the hijiki.)
6. Bring to the boil, cover, reduce the heat to low and simmer for 35 minutes.
7. Add the remaining 1 tablespoon shoyu and the sautéed onions and simmer for another 20-25 minutes until the liquid evaporates.
8. To prepare the rolls, place 2-3 tablespoons of the filling across each crêpe, carefully roll up each crepe and slice into 1½ inch (4cm) lengths.
9. Place on a serving tray in a decorative arrangement, garnished with chopped spring onions (scallions).

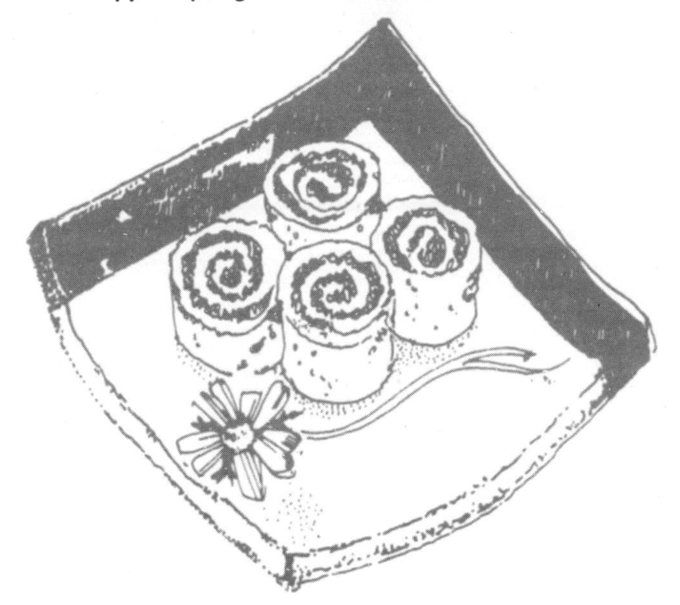

Hijiki with Almonds

Serves 4-5

Imperial (Metric)
1¾ oz (50g) hijiki
Water to cover hijiki
1½ tablespoons shoyu
2 oz (55g) roasted chopped almonds
Spring onions or parsley, to garnish

American
½ cup hijiki
Water to cover hijiki
1½ tablespoons shoyu
½ cup roasted chopped almonds
Scallions or parsley, to garnish

1. Wash and soak the hijiki as described on page 100. Remove and cut into 1½ inch (4cm) lengths.
2. Place the soaking water in a pot (except the last part which may contain fine sand particles). (If this soaking water tastes too salty, use half only and add fresh water to cover the hijiki.)
3. Add the hijiki, bring to the boil, cover, reduce the heat to low and simmer for 35 minutes.
4. Add the shoyu and cook for a further 20-25 minutes until the liquid has evaporated. Mix with the chopped roasted almonds and serve, garnished with spring onions (scallions) or parsley.

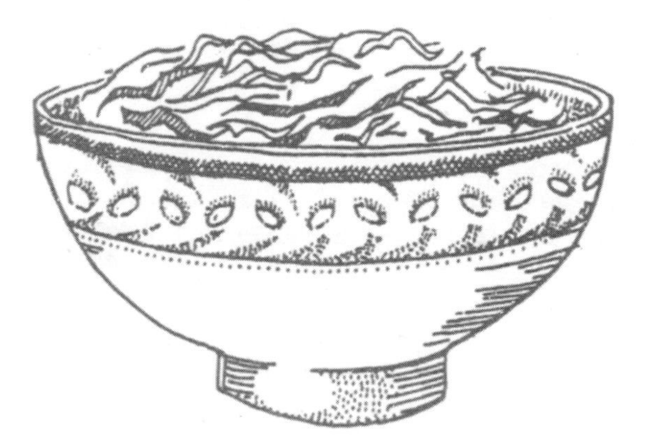

Hijiki Tofu Balls

Serves 4-5

Imperial (Metric)
6 oz (170g) tofu
¾ oz (20g) hijiki
Water to cover hijiki
½ tablespoon shoyu
3 oz (85g) chopped carrots
1½ oz (45g) chopped burdock
1½ oz (45g) sesame seeds, roasted
Pinch of sea salt
1½ oz (30g) wholemeal flour (optional)
Sesame oil for deep frying
Lettuce leaves to garnish

American
1 cup tofu
¼ cup hijiki
Water to cover hijiki
½ tablespoon shoyu
½ cup chopped carrots
¼ cup chopped burdock
¼ cup sesame seeds, roasted
Pinch of sea salt
¼ cup wholewheat flour (optional)
Sesame oil for deep frying
Lettuce leaves to garnish

1. Wrap the block of tofu in a absorbent cloth and place on a wooden cutting board. Put a weight or heavy plate on top to squeeze out excess liquid from the tofu. Leave for 20 minutes. Remove the weight and cloth and purée in a suribachi or bowl with a fork.
2. Wash and soak the hijiki (see page 100).
3. Place the soaking water in a pot (do not use the last part as this may contain small sand particles), add the hijiki, bring to the boil, cover, reduce the flame to low and simmer for 35 minutes. Add the shoyu and cook for a further 20-25 minutes until the liquid has evaporated.
4. Leave to cool for a while then cut the hijiki into very small pieces.
5. Mix together in a bowl the cooked hijiki, raw carrots, burdock, puréed tofu, sesame seeds and a pinch of sea salt. Shape into small balls, and if the consistency is too soft, add the wholewheat flour to bind.
6. Heat 2-3 inches of sesame oil in a pot to 350°F/180°C taking care to see it does not smoke. Drop the balls a few at a time into the oil and leave for 2-3 minutes. Turn over and cook for another 1-2 minutes until they become golden brown all over. Remove and place on a paper towel to drain.
7. Place the lettuce leaves on a serving plate and sit the balls on top. Serve hot with a dipping sauce of either fresh ginger juice, shoyu and water or grated daikon radish with a few drops of shoyu.

Hijiki with Sautéed Mixed Vegetables

Serves 5-6

Imperial (Metric)

1¾ oz (50g) hijiki
Water to cover hijiki
1 tablespoon shoyu
Few drops of sesame oil
6 oz (170g) onions, cut in half moons
3 oz (85g) carrots, cut in matchsticks
Pinch of sea salt
2 oz (55g) white cabbage, finely cut into 4 inch (10cm) long strips
3 oz (85g) seitan wheat gluten, cut in matchsticks
Spring onions, to garnish

American

½ cup hijiki
Water to cover hijiki
1 tablespoon shoyu
Few drops of sesame oil
1 cup onions, cut in half moons
½ cup carrots, cut in matchsticks
Pinch of sea salt
½ cup white cabbage, finely cut into 4 inch long strips
½ cup seitan wheat meat, cut in matchsticks
Scallions, to garnish

1. Wash and soak the hijiki (see page 100). Remove (keeping the soaking water) and slice into 1½ inch (4cm) long pieces.
2. Place the soaking water in a pot (except the last part which may contain small sand particles). If the soaking water tastes too salty use half only and top up to cover the hijiki with fresh water. Add the hijiki, bring to the boil, cover, reduce the heat to low and simmer for 35 minutes.
3. Add the shoyu and cook for a further 20 minutes until the liquid has evaporated.
4. Lightly brush a frying pan with sesame oil and heat. Sauté the onions uncovered for 5-7 minutes. Add the carrots and a pinch of sea salt and sauté for 2-3 minutes more.
5. Add the white cabbage and seitan and sauté for a further 3-4 minutes. During all the sautéing stir the vegetables constantly to avoid burning and ensure even cooking.
6. Add the hijiki to the vegetables and sauté together for 2-3 minutes.
7. Place in a serving dish and garnish with the chopped spring onions (scallions).

Note: Any variety of seasonal vegetables can be used in this dish.

Hijiki Summer Salad

Serves 4-6

Imperial (Metric)	American
1¾ oz (50g) hijiki	½ cup hijiki
Water to cover hijiki	Water to cover hijiki
1 tablespoon shoyu	1 tablespoon shoyu
Pinch of sea salt	Pinch of sea salt
3 fresh cobs of corn	3 fresh ears of corn
3 oz (85g) shelled green peas	½ cup shelled green peas
2 oz (55g) beansprouts	½ cup beansprouts
3 oz (85g) grated carrots	½ cup grated carrots
Dressing:	*Dressing:*
4 tablespoons natural mustard	4 tablespoons natural mustard
2 tablespoons sesame spread	2 tablespoons sesame butter
3 tablespoons brown rice vinegar	3 tablespoons brown rice vinegar
3 tablespoons water	3 tablespoons water

1. Wash and soak the hijiki (see page 100). Remove (keeping the soaking water) and slice into 1½ inch (4cm) lengths.
2. Place the soaking water in a pot (discarding the last part which may contain small sand particles). If this soaking water tastes too salty use half only and top up with fresh water to cover the hijiki. Bring to the boil, cover, reduce the heat to low and simmer for 35 minutes.
3. Add the shoyu and cook for a further 20-25 minutes until the water has evaporated.
4. Bring a pot of water to the boil, add a pinch of sea salt and the cobs of corn and cook for 20 minutes until soft. Remove the corn kernels from the cobs. In the same water boil the peas for 10 minutes, and then the beansprouts for 2-3 minutes, placing each on a plate to cool after cooking.
5. In a serving bowl mix together the cooked hijiki, green peas, beansprouts, raw grated carrot and the cooked corn kernels.
6. Blend all the dressing ingredients together until they become smooth, then add to the salad and mix well before serving.

Vinegared Hijiki

Serves 3-4

Imperial (Metric)	American
1¾ oz (50g) hijiki	½ cup hijiki
Water to cover hijiki	Water to cover hijiki
1 tablespoon shoyu	1 tablespoon shoyu
4 tablespoons brown rice vinegar	4 tablespoons brown rice vinegar
1½ oz (45g) mustard cress or watercress	3 cups mustard cress or watercress

1. Wash and soak the hijiki (see page 100). Remove (keeping the soaking water) and cut into 1½ inch (4cm) lengths.
2. Place the soaking water in a pot (leaving the last part which may contain small sand particles). If this soaking water tastes too salty, use half only and top up to cover the hijiki with fresh water. Add the hijiki, bring to the boil, cover, reduce the heat to low and simmer for 35 minutes.
3. Add the shoyu and brown rice vinegar and cook for a further 20-25 minutes until the liquid has evaporated.
4. Mix the mustard cress or watercress in with the cooked hijiki and serve.

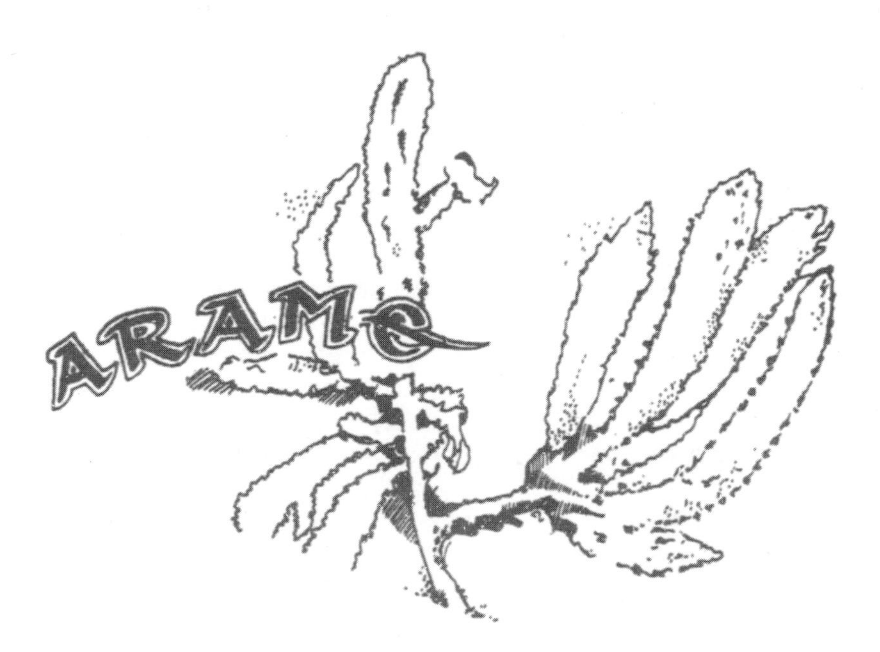

Although superficially resembling hijiki, arame is quite a different vegetable with a softer texture and a milder and sweeter flavour. It is one of the oriental sea vegetables that is usually readily acceptable to the western palate. Its light taste harmonizes well with tofu and more delicate tasting land vegetables, and it makes an attractive dish cooked and served with a vinegar and shoyu marinade.

Arame is a member of the brown group of algae and is mainly harvested around the famous Ise peninsula on the Pacific side of Japan's main island. The plants consist of wavy strips of fronds each about twelve inches (15cm) long and one and a half (4cm) inches wide. Arame inhabits the rocks below the lower water line and was traditionally harvested by hand by women divers. The fronds are inherently tough and like hijiki they are boiled for several hours to soften, and at the same time deepen, their colour. To allow for easier cooking and use, the fronds are usually sliced into thin thread-like strips giving a superficial appearance similar to hijiki. Arame requires a brief soaking before cooking, during which time its volume will almost double.

Arame's sweet taste derives from its high content of the natural non-caloric sugar, mannitol, which is present in many brown algae. Along with kombu and hijiki, arame's balance of minerals can counteract high blood-pressure and it has also been used as a traditional folk remedy for treating disorders of the female reproductive organs. Like other brown sea vegetables, arame is especially rich in iodine and calcium.

Note that the best method of washing and soaking arame is to place it in a bowl, cover with water and stir around. Then put the arame in a second bowl and repeat with fresh water. Repeat again, this time using a cooking pot, and the correct amount of water for soaking, as stated in the recipe.

Stuffed Pumpkin with Arame

Serves 5-6

Imperial (Metric)	American
1 medium pumpkin (4 lbs/1.8k)	1 medium winter squash (4 pounds)
Pinch of sea salt	Pinch of sea salt
1¾ oz (50g) arame	1 cup arame
Water to cover arame	Water to cover arame
2 tablespoons shoyu	2 tablespoons shoyu
Few drops of sesame oil	Few drops of sesame oil
9 oz (255g) onions, diced	1½ cups onions, diced
2½ oz (70g) fresh mushrooms, finely sliced	1 cup fresh mushrooms, finely sliced
½ oz (15g) chopped parsley	½ cup chopped parsley
4 oz (115g) cooked couscous	1 cup cooked couscous

1. Slice the top off the pumpkin (squash), set to one side, then remove the seeds and centre.
2. Sprinkle a few grains of sea salt inside the pumpkin and then steam with the top in a basket or in a pan filled with 1 inch (2.5cm) of water until the flesh is cooked. Place in a serving bowl.
3. Wash and soak the arame (see above).
4. Place the soaking water in a pot (discarding the last part which may contain small sand particles). Add the arame, bring to the boil, cover, reduce the heat to low and simmer for 20 minutes. Add 1 tablespoon of the shoyu and cook for a further 10 minutes until the liquid has evaporated.
5. Lightly brush a frying pan with sesame oil, heat, and sauté the onions for 5-7 minutes. Add the mushrooms and the other tablespoon of shoyu and sauté for a further 5-7 minutes. Add the parsley, cooked arame and couscous, mix well and turn off the heat.

6. Fill the pumpkin with the cooked arame mix, replace the top of the pumpkin, and serve.

Note: If you wish to serve the pumpkin hot, place in a warm oven for 5 minutes.

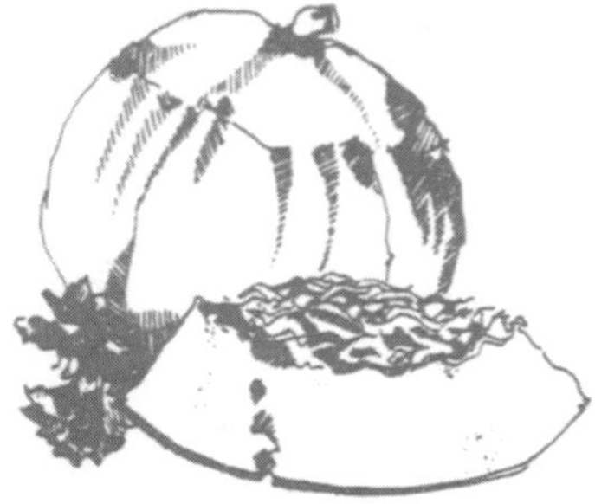

Arame with Deep Fried Tofu

Serves 2-3

Imperial (Metric)	American
½ lb (225g) block of tofu	½ pound block of tofu
Arrowroot	Arrowroot
Sesame oil for deep frying	Sesame oil for deep frying
1¾ oz (50g) arame	1 cup arame
Water to cover arame	Water to cover arame
½ tablespoon shoyu	½ tablespoon shoyu
2 bunches watercress, cut into 1 inch (2.5cm) lengths	2 bunches watercress, cut into 1 inch lengths

1. Wrap the tofu in a tea towel and place on a wooden cutting board. Place a weight or plate on top and leave for 20 minutes to press out the excess liquid. Uncover the tofu and slice into small rectangles about ½ inch × 1 inch (1cm × 2.5cm). Lightly coat each piece with arrowroot.
2. Heat about 2 inches (5cm) of sesame oil in a pot to 350°F/180°C and deep fry the tofu until it is golden brown all over. Remove from the oil and place on a paper towel to drain.
3. Wash and soak the arame (see page 108).
4. Place the soaking water in a pot (discarding the last part which may contain small sand particles). Add the arame, bring to the boil, cover, reduce the heat to low and simmer for 20 minutes.
5. Add the shoyu and fried tofu and cook for a further 10 minutes until the liquid has evaporated. Add the watercress and mix in well.
6. Place in a bowl and serve.

Arame Tempeh Salad

Serves 2-3

Imperial (Metric)
½ lb (225g) tempeh
1¾ oz (50g) arame
Water to cover arame
2 tablespoons shoyu
Pinch of sea salt
5 oz (140g) carrots, cut into matchsticks
1 bunch red radishes, cut into quarters

Dressing:
3 tablespoons natural mustard
3 tablespoons water or pickle juice

American
½ pound block of tempeh
1 cup arame
Water to cover arame
2 tablespoons shoyu
Pinch of sea salt
1 cup carrots, cut into matchsticks
1 bunch red radishes, cut into quarters

Dressing:
3 tablespoons natural mustard
3 tablespoons water or pickle juice

1. If the tempeh has been deep frozen, make sure it has thoroughly defrosted before using. Cut the tempeh into 1 inch (2.5cm) squares.
2. Wash and soak the arame (see page 108).
3. Place the soaking water in a pot (discarding the last part which may contain small sand particles). Add the arame and tempeh, bring to the boil, cover, reduce the heat to low and simmer for 20 minutes. Add the shoyu and cook for a further 10 minutes until the liquid has evaporated.
4. Bring a pot of water to the boil. Add a pinch of sea salt and boil the carrots for 2-3 minutes. Remove and place on a plate to cool. Repeat, using the same cooking water for the radishes, but cook for only ½ minute.
5. In a serving bowl mix together the arame, tempeh, carrots and radishes.
6. Mix the dressing ingredients together and pour over the salad.

Arame Chinese Cabbage Leaf Rolls

Serves 3-4

Imperial (Metric)	American
5 large Chinese cabbage leaves	5 large Chinese cabbage leaves
Pinch of sea salt	Pinch of sea salt
1¾ oz (50g) arame	1 cup arame
Water to cover arame	Water to cover arame
1½ tablespoons shoyu	1½ tablespoons shoyu

1. Bring a pot of water to the boil, add a pinch of sea salt and quickly boil the Chinese cabbage leaves for ½ minute. Remove and place on a plate to cool.
2. Wash and soak the arame (see page 108).
3. Place the soaking water in a pot (discarding the last part which may contain small sand particles). Add the arame, bring to the boil, cover, reduce the heat to low and simmer for 20 minutes. Add the shoyu and cook for a further 10 minutes until the liquid has evaporated.
4. Carefully spread out one cabbage leaf at a time on a cutting board and evenly place one fifth of the cooked arame on top. Firmly roll up the leaf, pressing it together to form a firm log. Cut the roll in half across the centre. Repeat for the other 4 cabbage leaves. If necessary, secure the rolls with a cocktail stick.
5. Place the cut rolls ends upward on a flat serving dish.

Note: These light green and black rolls make an attractive and colourful dish. They are especially useful 'finger foods' for parties, picnics and for travelling.

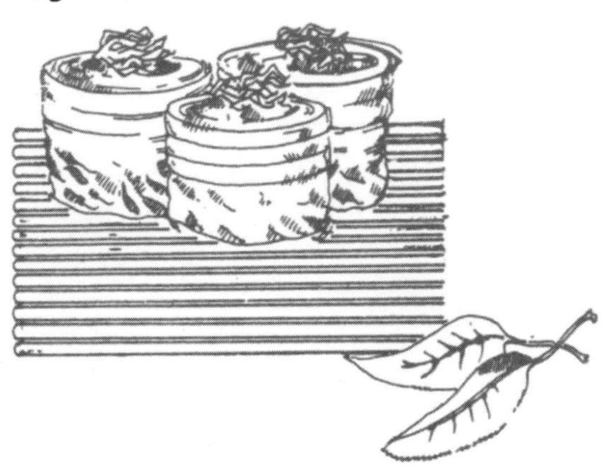

Arame with Broccoli and Mushrooms

See front cover photograph
Serves 3-4

Imperial (Metric)	American
1¾ oz (50g) arame	1 cup arame
Water to cover arame	Water to cover arame
5 oz (140g) fresh mushrooms, sliced	2 cups fresh mushrooms, sliced
1½ tablespoons shoyu	1½ tablespoons shoyu
Pinch of sea salt	Pinch of sea salt
5 oz (140g) broccoli, cut into small florets	1 cup broccoli, cut into small florets

1. Wash and soak the arame (see page 108).
2. Place the soaking water in a pot (discarding the last part which may contain small sand particles). Add the arame, cover, reduce the heat to low and simmer for 20 minutes. Add the mushrooms and shoyu and cook for a further 10 minutes until the liquid has evaporated.
3. In another pot, bring some water to the boil, add a pinch of sea salt and the broccoli and cook for 2-3 minutes. Remove and leave on plate to cool.
4. Mix the broccoli together with the arame and mushrooms in a serving bowl.

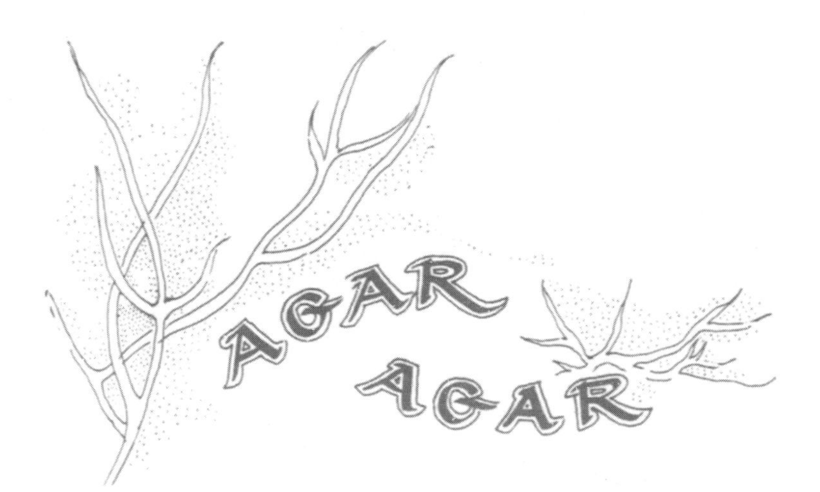

Agar-agar, known as kanten in Japan, is a wonderful natural gelatine that has a very mild flavour, yet is nutritionally rich containing a wealth of minerals. It can be used to make delicious dessert jellies and savoury aspics, as its neutral taste will not interfere with the natural flavour of fruits and vegetables.

Agar-agar produces a firmer gel than commercial gelatine and will not melt so readily. It is also completely vegetarian and free of calories. For a refreshing light dessert on a hot summer day the cooling effect of a fruit kanten is hard to beat, and in winter a stronger flavoured savoury aspic will add a light touch to a nourishing meal. Agar-agar is quick and easy to prepare requiring just a brief cooking, but remember to allow a good hour for setting at room temperature.

Agar-agar is prepared from the gelidium species of red sea vegetables, known as *tengusa* in Japan, whose cell walls contain an abundance of complex polysaccharide starches somewhat similar to cellulose. In their wild form they are strongly flavoured and somewhat foul tasting and processing is necessary to dissolve the starchy fibres and neutralize their taste. There are two ways that this can be achieved. Firstly, the modern commercial way involves the use of sulphuric acid to dissolve the starches, and inorganic bleaches and dyes to neutralize the colour and flavour. Most powder agar-agar is prepared this way, as are many of the thread or bar agar-agars found in oriental stores. These are of poor quality and are all best avoided. The second way is to process in the time-honoured traditional manner. The sea vegetables are gathered and dried on the shore. They are then transported into the mountains in winter where they are cooked down with a little mild vinegar to soften the coarse fibres. The thick soupy mix which results is then pressed through cloth expelling a smooth liquid. This is poured into large tray-like moulds and left to set. The gelatin is then sliced into bars which are placed outside on low bamboo frames positioned to gain the maximum amount of sunlight. Over a period of a week or two the cold temperatures at night freeze the bars and each day the sun melts them, eliminating their water content, until all that is left is a very lightweight dry fibrous bar of starch that has been naturally bleached to a light grey colour and has had its flavour neutralized. (The Japanese name *kanten* means cold sky.) These bars are then packaged whole, or more commonly nowadays, cut into fine flakes to save space and expense in shipping. Flake or bar agar-agar made by this traditional method is the type sold by most quality-conscious health and natural food stores. It is more expensive than the powdered commercial product, but is a genuine natural food and the type we recommend for use. Natural agar-agar is rich in iodine and trace minerals and has long been recognized for its mildly laxative properties, which can be further enhanced by the addition of fresh ginger juice.

The gelling ability of natural agar-agar varies according to the acidity or alkalinity of the food with which it is used. Acid foods often require more agar-agar than alkaline foods. Also, being a natural product, you may find that each batch of agar-agar has a different potency and your personal taste may be for a firmer or softer gel. For these reasons the amount of agar-agar indicated in our recipes is only a guide. If you wish to check the gel take a small spoonful of the heated mix and place it on a cold surface to set. This will only take a minute or two. You can then adjust if required by adding more agar-agar or more liquid to the pot. Our recipes use natural agar-agar flakes, as these are commonly available. Usually one cup of flakes with five cups of liquid will produce an adequate gel. If you are using natural agar-agar bars first break the bars into small pieces and soak for one hour. Squeeze out the excess liquid then proceed as indicated for the flakes. One bar of natural agar-agar with 2 cups of liquid is the standard ratio to achieve a suitable gel.

Note: As natural agar-agar flakes are usually sold in 28g packets, 1 oz is translated in this chapter as 28g (not 30g).

Noodle Kanten

Serves 4-5

Imperial (Metric)	American
4 oz (115g) (dry weight) udon noodles or wholewheat noodles, cooked	4 ounces (dry weight) udon noodles or wholewheat noodles, cooked
3 oz (85g) chopped spring onions	1 cup chopped scallions
1¼ pints (700ml) water	3 cups water
½ oz (14g) agar-agar flakes	½ cup agar-agar flakes
2 fl oz (60ml) shoyu	¼ cup shoyu
½ carrot, sliced thinly	½ carrot, sliced thinly

1. Cut the cooked noodles into approximately 2 inch (5cm) lengths and place in a rinsed shallow dish or mould with the chopped spring onions (scallions).
2. In a pot, add the water and the agar-agar flakes and leave to soak for 10-15 minutes. Then bring to the boil, reduce the heat and stirring constantly, simmer for a few minutes until the flakes have dissolved. Add the shoyu.
3. Pour the liquid over the noodles making sure they are completely covered. Place the sliced carrots on top.
4. Leave to cool until firm, then cut into small squares, triangles or other shapes and arrange attractively on a tray to serve.

Note: It is important to rinse the dish or mould before adding the liquid so the kanten can be easily removed.

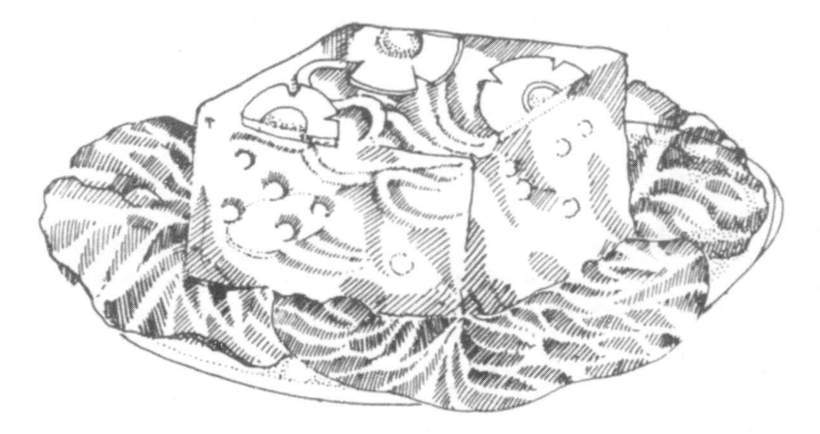

Tofu Kanten

Serves 4-5

Imperial (Metric)	American
½ lb (225g) tofu	½ pound block of tofu
1¼ pints (700ml) water	3 cups water
½ oz (14g) agar-agar flakes	½ cup agar-agar flakes
2 fl oz (60ml) umeboshi vinegar	¼ cup umeboshi vinegar
6 oz (170g) cucumber, diced	1 cup cucumber, diced
Spring onions, chopped, to garnish (optional)	Scallions, chopped, to garnish (optional)

1. Crumble the tofu in a suribachi or with a fork.
2. Place the water in a pot, add the agar-agar flakes and leave to soak for 10-15 minutes. Bring to the boil, reduce the heat and simmer for a few minutes, stirring constantly, until the flakes are completely dissolved. Add the tofu and umeboshi vinegar and simmer for a further 2-3 minutes. Add the cucumber at the end.
3. Rinse a shallow dish or mould and pour in the mix. Leave to cool until firm. Cut into desired shapes and serve. Garnish with chopped spring onions (scallions) if desired.

Aduki Raisin Kanten

Serves 4-5

Imperial (Metric)	American
8 oz (225g) aduki beans	½ cup aduki beans
1 strip of kombu, 2½ inches (6cm) long	1 strip of kombu, 2½ inches long
2½ pints (1.4 litres) water	6 cups water
9 oz (255g) raisins	1½ cups raisins
¼ teaspoon sea salt	¼ teaspoon sea salt
½-¾ oz (14-20g) agar-agar flakes	½-¾ cup agar-agar flakes

1. Place the aduki beans, kombu and water in a heavy pot and leave to soak for 4-5 hours. Heat and bring to the boil, then cover and simmer on a low heat for 45 minutes.
2. Add the raisins and continue cooking for a further 30 minutes or until the aduki beans are tender.
3. Add the sea salt and cook for 15-20 minutes more.
4. Soak the agar-agar flakes in half a cup of water for 10-15 minutes.

Add the flakes and soaking water to the pot of aduki beans and simmer for a few minutes until the flakes have completely dissolved.

3. Rinse a shallow dish or mould, pour in the aduki mixture and leave to cool until firm. Cut into desired shapes and serve. Aduki raisin kanten makes a rich and sweet dessert.

Variation: This dish can also be prepared with the addition of chopped roasted nuts. They should be added just before adding the mix to the setting dish.

Couscous Apricot Kanten

Serves 4-5

Imperial (Metric)	American
6 oz (170g) cooked couscous	1½ cups cooked couscous
10 oz (285g) dried apricots	2 cups dried apricots
2½ pints (1.4 litres) water	6 cups water
Pinch of sea salt	Pinch of sea salt
1 oz (28g) agar-agar flakes	1 cup agar-agar flakes

1. Spread the cooked couscous evenly in a rinsed shallow dish or mould.
2. Rinse the apricots under cold water to clean, then place in a pot with 5 cups of the water and a pinch of sea salt. Bring to the boil and simmer gently for 30 minutes.
3. Soak the agar-agar flakes in the remaining cup of water for 10-15 minutes. Add to the apricots and simmer for a few minutes, stirring constantly, until the flakes have completely dissolved.
4. Pour the mix gently over the couscous and leave to cool until firm. Cut into desired shapes and serve.

Variation: Other dried fruits can be used instead of apricots. Fresh seasonal fruits can also be used but will only need cooking for a few minutes. This dish can be decorated with chopped, roasted nuts if desired.

Chestnut Kanten

Serves 4-5

Imperial (Metric)	American
½ lb (225g) dried chestnuts	1 cup dried chestnuts
1¼ pints (700ml) water	3 cups water
1 strip of kombu, 3 inches (7.5cm) long	1 strip of kombu, 3 inches long
1 pint (570ml) apple juice	2½ cups apple juice
¼ teaspoon sea salt	¼ teaspoon sea salt
¾ oz (20g) agar-agar flakes	¾ cup agar-agar flakes
Thin slices of orange to decorate	Thin slices of orange to decorate

1. Soak the chestnuts overnight in the water.
2. Add the kombu and 2 cups of the apple juice and bring to the boil. Reduce the heat and cook for 1 hour or until the chestnuts are tender.
3. Add the sea salt and cook for a further 15-20 minutes.
4. Purée the chestnuts in a suribachi or with a hand food mill.
5. Soak the agar-agar flakes in the remaining apple juice for 10-15 minutes. Combine with the chestnut purée and simmer for a few minutes, stirring constantly, until the flakes have completely dissolved.
5. Rinse a shallow dish or mould, pour in the mixture and leave to cool until firm. Cut into desired shapes and serve, decorated on top with half a thin slice of orange.

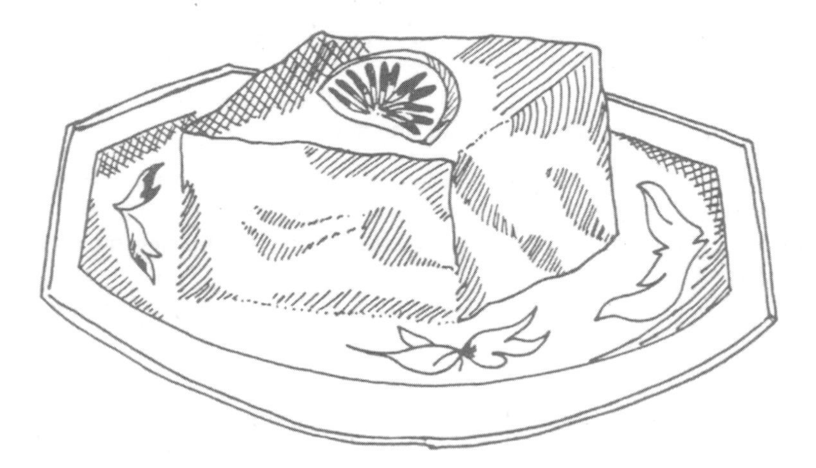

Strawberry Kanten

See back cover photograph
Serves 4-5

Imperial (Metric)	American
½ lb (225g) fresh strawberries	½ pound fresh strawberries
Pinch of sea salt	Pinch of sea salt
8 fl oz (230ml) water	1 cup water
1¼ pints (700ml) apple juice	3 cups apple juice
½-¾ oz (14-20g) agar-agar flakes	½-¾ cup agar-agar flakes
4 tablespoons barley malt	4 tablespoons barley malt

1. Wash the strawberries carefully and cut in half. Place in a bowl, add a pinch of sea salt and leave for ½ hour to bring out their sweetness.
2. To a pot, add the water, apple juice and agar-agar flakes and leave to soak for 10-15 minutes. Bring to the boil, reduce the heat, add the barley malt (taste the mix — if not sweet enough, add more) and simmer for a few minutes, stirring constantly, until the flakes have completely dissolved.
3. Add the strawberries to the cooked liquid, then place this mixture in a rinsed shallow dish or mould. Leave to cool until firm. Cut in desired shapes and serve, topping each shape with half a strawberry if desired.

Note: Depending on the sweetness of your strawberries, you may need to use more or less barley malt. Check the taste of your strawberries first, then if required, adjust the amount of barley malt when it is added to the cooked liquid.

Apple Sesame Custard

Serves 4-5

Imperial (Metric)	American
2½ pints (1.4 litres) apple juice	6 cups apple juice
1 oz (28g) agar-agar flakes	1 cup agar-agar flakes
2 tablespoons natural vanilla extract	2 tablespoons natural vanilla extract
3 tablespoons finely grated lemon peel	3 tablespoons finely grated lemon peel
5 tablespoons sesame spread or tahini	5 tablespoons sesame butter or tahini
Pinch of sea salt	Pinch of sea salt

1. Place the apple juice and agar-agar flakes in a pot and leave to soak for 10-15 minutes. Bring to the boil, reduce the heat and simmer for a few minutes, stirring constantly, until the flakes have all dissolved.
2. With a little of the hot liquid, mix together the vanilla extract, grated lemon peel, sesame spread (sesame butter) or tahini and sea salt into a creamy consistency. Add to the hot liquid.
3. Rinse a shallow dish or mould in water and then pour in the hot liquid and leave to cool until firm.
4. Place in a blender and purée until smooth. Serve on its own or as a topping for desserts.

Note: This is a very refreshing dessert, especially on a hot day if it is served after being chilled in a refrigerator.

Tangerine Kanten

See back cover photograph

Imperial (Metric)	American
Large tangerines or medium oranges, enough to produce ¾ pint (425ml) of juice	Large tangerines or medium oranges, enough to produce 2 cups of juice
½ oz (14g) agar-agar flakes	½ cup agar-agar flakes
¼ pint (140ml) water	⅔ cup water
Few grains of sea salt	Few grains of sea salt
2½ tablespoons barley malt	2½ tablespoons barley malt

1. Carefully cut the tangerines or oranges so that they look like little baskets (see below and back cover photograph), removing the inner pulp and squeezing out the juice.
2. Soak the agar-agar in the water for 10-15 minutes. Add the tangerine or orange juice, bring to the boil, reduce the heat to low, add the sea salt and barley malt and simmer for a few minutes until the flakes have completely dissolved.
3. Pour some of the kanten mix into each tangerine or orange basket and leave until it becomes firm. Arrange the baskets attractively on a tray.

Note: Alternatively, the kanten can be set in a dish and then cut into squares and placed in the baskets. The back cover photograph shows this presentation.

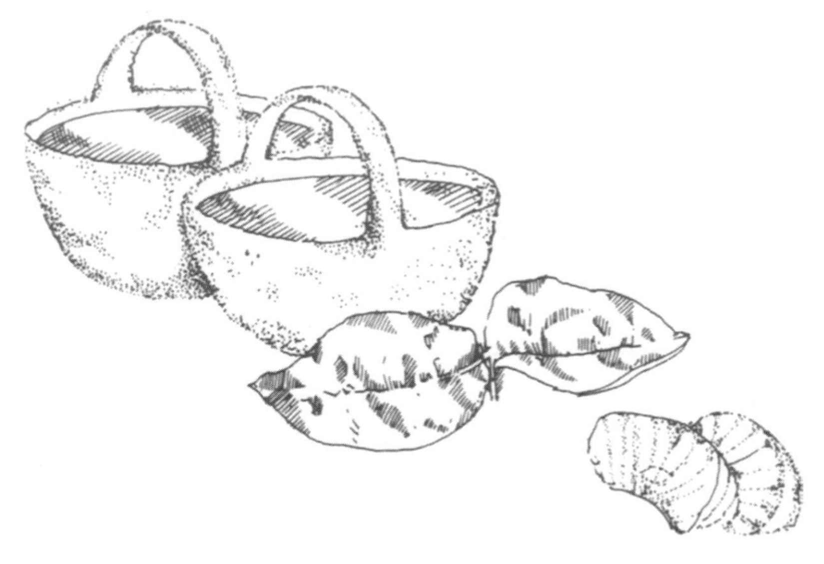

Almond Jelly

Serves 4-5

Imperial (Metric)	American
1 oz (28g) agar-agar flakes	1 cup agar-agar flakes
3 pints (1.7 litres) pear juice	7½ cups pear juice
6 tablespoons barley malt	6 tablespoons barley malt
Pinch of sea salt	Pinch of sea salt
2 tablespoons juice from freshly grated ginger root	2 tablespoons juice from freshly grated ginger root
4 oz (115g) roasted chopped almonds	1 cup roasted chopped almonds

1. Soak the agar-agar flakes in the pear juice for 10-15 minutes.
2. Bring to the boil in a pan, reduce the heat, add the barley malt and a pinch of sea salt and cook, stirring constantly, for a few minutes until the flakes have completely dissolved.
3. Add the fresh ginger juice.
4. Rinse a shallow dish or mould in water, pour in the liquid mixture and leave to cool until almost firm. Stir vigorously, chill again, stir once more, add the chopped roasted almonds and serve.

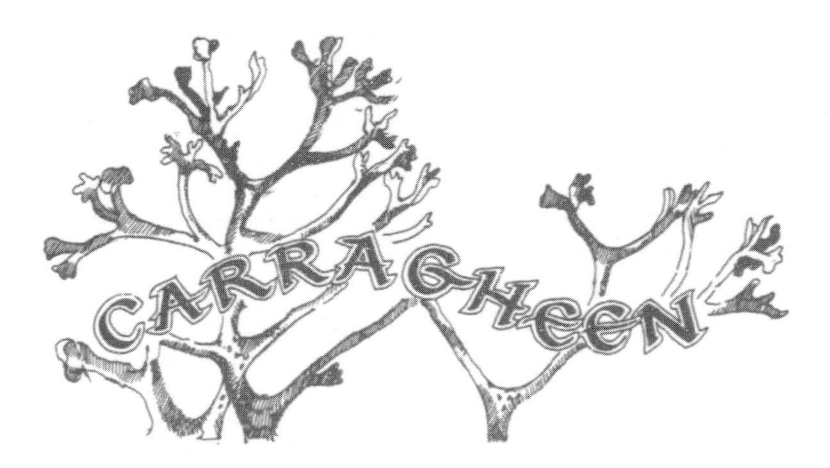

Carragheen, like agar-agar, has been used for centuries for its gelling properties. It makes a softer gel than agar-agar and is more commonly used as a thickener for soups, stews and sauces, where its mineral-rich taste adds a characteristic flavour to the dish.

Carragheen is also known as *Irish moss,* and although it is found abundantly around the Emerald Isle, it also frequents the temperate waters on both sides of the Atlantic. It is a small bush-like plant with dense reddish purple fronds growing between six and twelve inches (15-30cm) long in a carpet on the rocks around the low water line. The fronds are carefully hand picked during the late summer, leaving the holdfasts secure for future growth. The fronds are first washed in salt water to remove any sand and then left to dry in the sun and wind for about ten days, during which time they will either partially or completely bleach to a silvery white. As with dulse, which comes from a similar shoreline habitat, carragheen should be carefully sorted before cooking to clean out any remaining shell pieces.

The gelling ability of carragheen, as with agar-agar, derives from a high content of polysaccharide starches known as *carrageenin.* Medicinally carragheen has a reputation as a healer of diarrhoea, urinary disorders and chronic chest infections. The plants themselves resemble the structure of the lungs, and traditionally a thick drink of carragheen with lemon and a natural sweetener has been used as a respiratory tonic. During the Second World War when the people of the Channel Islands were short of food, they ate ample quantities of their local carragheen and there was a marked decrease in the number of colds and bronchial infections. Carragheen is rich in minerals, especially iodine, and contains a good supply of vitamin A.

Unlike agar-agar, carragheen is unprocessed, and a proportionally larger amount needs to be used, which must be briefly soaked and well cooked to produce a gel. A light cooking will leave it as a tasty vegetable, but if you require it fully dissolved, you will need to cook longer, having first sorted and discarded the coarser parts of the plant. The thickening ability of carragheen may vary according to its origin and the time of harvest. The amounts indicated in the recipes should only be used as a rough guide.

Carragheen Miso Soup

Serves 3-4

Imperial (Metric)	American
½ oz (15g) carragheen	½ cup carragheen
2½ pints (1.4 litres) water	6 cups water
3 oz (85g) pumpkin, diced	½ cup winter squash, diced
1 medium onion, diced	1 medium onion, diced
2 tablespoons barley (mugi) miso	2 tablespoons barley (mugi) miso
Parsley, chopped, to garnish	Parsley, chopped, to garnish

1. Thoroughly sort the carragheen, removing any shell particles or foreign matter. Rinse quickly several times to clean.
2. Place the carragheen in a pot with the water and soak for 30 minutes.
3. Bring to the boil, reduce the flames and simmer for 1 hour or more until the carragheen has almost dissolved. Stir occasionally to prevent sticking.
4. Add the pumpkin (winter squash) and onion and cook uncovered for 10-15 minutes until soft.
5. Purée the miso with a little of the soup liquid, then add to the pot and simmer for 2 minutes over a very low heat.
6. Garnish with chopped parsley.

Note: If the soup becomes too thick after cooking the carragheen, add more water before adding the vegetables.

Celery Soup

Serves 3-4

Imperial (Metric)	American
½ oz (15g) carragheen	½ cup carragheen
2½ pints (1.4 litres) water	6 cups water
2½ oz (70g) leeks, finely sliced diagonally	½ cup leeks, finely sliced diagonally
4 oz (115g) celery, finely sliced diagonally	1 cup celery, finely diced diagonally
2 tablespoons barley (mugi) miso	2 tablespoons barley (mugi) miso

1. Wash the carragheen and remove any small stones, then rinse quickly several times. Place in a pot with the water and soak for 30 minutes.
2. Bring to the boil, reduce the flame and simmer for 1 hour or more until the carragheen has almost dissolved. Stir occasionally to prevent sticking.
3. Add the leeks and celery and cook uncovered for 10 minutes.
4. Purée the miso with a little of the soup liquid. Add to the soup and simmer for 2 minutes over a very low heat.
5. Garnish with small leaves from the celery.

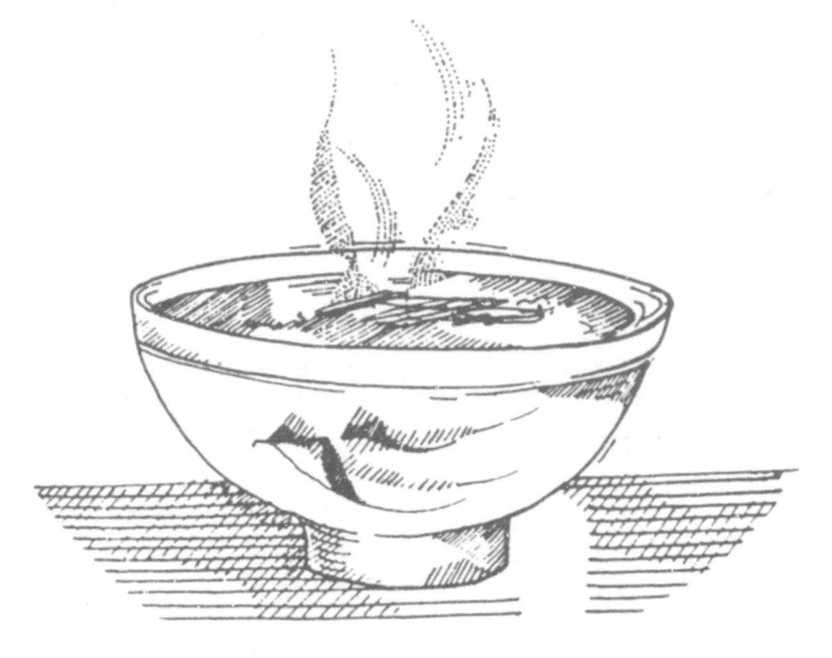

Spaghetti with Mushroom Sauce

Serves 2-3

Imperial (Metric)	American
1¼ pints (700ml) water	3 cups water
Pinch of sea salt	Pinch of sea salt
½ lb (225g) wholewheat spaghetti	½ pound wholewheat spaghetti
¼ oz (7g) carragheen	¼ cup carragheen
Few drops of sesame oil (preferably roasted)	Few drops of sesame oil (preferably roasted)
9 oz (255g) onions, diced	1½ cups onions, diced
2½ oz (70g) fresh mushrooms, cut finely	1 cup fresh mushrooms, cut finely
2 tablespoons shoyu	2 tablespoons shoyu
1 oz (30g) chopped, roasted almonds	¼ cup chopped, roasted almonds
Chopped spring onions to garnish	Chopped scallions to garnish

1. Bring the water to the boil, add a pinch of sea salt and the spaghetti and return to the boil. Reduce the flame to medium low and cook until done (when the inside and outside of each spaghetti strand are the same colour). Place in a strainer and rinse under cold water to prevent sticking.
2. Clean and sort out small stones from the carragheen and rinse quickly several times. Place in a pot with the water and soak for 30 minutes. Bring to the boil and simmer for 1 hour or more until the carragheen has almost dissolved. Stir occasionally to prevent sticking.
3. Lightly oil a frying pan and heat. Add the onions and sauté for 5-6 minutes. Add the mushrooms and sauté for a further 6-7 minutes. Add the shoyu and simmer for 5 minutes.
4. Mix the carragheen sauce with the sautéed vegetables and chopped almonds and pour on top of the spaghetti. Garnish with chopped spring onions (scallions).

Winter Stew

Serves 3-4

Imperial (Metric)	American
½ oz (15g) carragheen	½ cup carragheen
1½ pints (850ml) water	3¾ cups water
1 oz (30g) burdock, cut in fine matchsticks	¼ cup burdock, cut in fine matchsticks
3 oz (85g) swede, cut in squares	½ cup rutabaga, cut in squares
2½ oz (70g) turnips, quartered	½ cup turnips, quartered
5 oz (140g) Brussels sprouts	1 cup Brussels sprouts
3 oz (85g) seitan wheat gluten, cut in squares	½ cup seitan wheat meat, cut in squares
3 oz (85g) tofu, cut in squares	½ cup tofu, cut in squares
3 tablespoons shoyu	3 tablespoons shoyu
2 tablespoons juice from freshly grated ginger root	2 tablespoons juice from freshly grated ginger root

1. Clean and sort out any small stones from the carragheen and rinse quickly several times. Place in a pot with the water and soak for 30 minutes.
2. Bring to the boil, reduce the heat and simmer for 1 hour or more until the carragheen has almost dissolved. Stir occasionally to prevent sticking.
3. In a heavy pot place in layers, the burdock, swede (rutabaga), turnips, Brussels sprouts, seitan and tofu. Season with the shoyu, add ¾ pint/425ml (2 cups) water and simmer for 20 minutes.
4. Add the carragheen sauce and ginger juice and simmer for 2 minutes before serving.

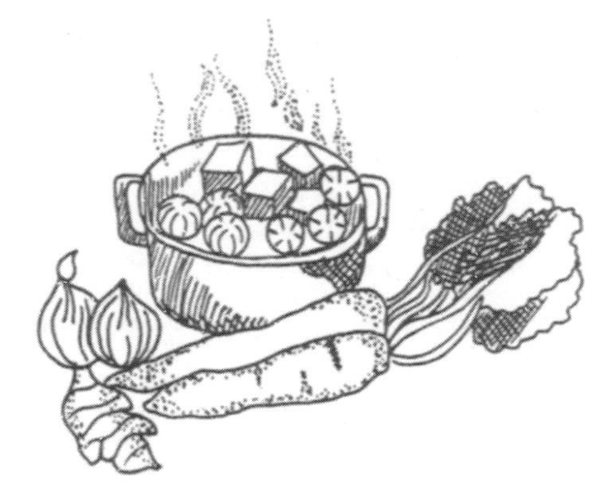

Onion Chrysanthemums

Serves 2

Imperial (Metric)	American
¼ oz (7g) carragheen	¼ cup carragheen
4 medium onions, peeled	4 medium onions, peeled
Pinch of sea salt	Pinch of sea salt
1 teaspoon brown rice (genmai) miso	1 teaspoon brown rice (genmai) miso
1¼ pints (700ml) water	3 cups water
Chopped parsley to garnish	Chopped parsley to garnish

1. Clean and sort out small stones from the carragheen and rinse quickly several times. Place the carragheen in a pot with the water and soak for 30 minutes.
2. Bring to the boil, reduce the heat and simmer for 1 hour or more until the carragheen has almost dissolved. Stir occasionally to prevent sticking.
3. Make four cuts in opposite directions across the top of each onion, cutting about two thirds down the onion each time.
4. Place the onions in a pot containing only ¼ inch (5mm) of water. Add a pinch of sea salt and simmer for 5 minutes.
5. Add the carragheen sauce.
6. Purée the miso with a small amount of the cooked liquid, put on top of the onions, cover and simmer for 10 minutes.
7. Garnish with chopped parsley.

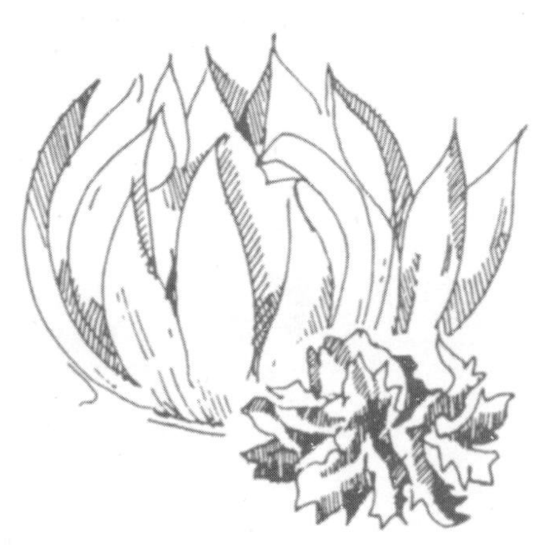

Multi-coloured Salad

Serves 2-3

Imperial (Metric)
½ oz (15g) carragheen
1¼ pints (700ml) water
Pinch of sea salt
2 medium carrots, sliced thinly
6 oz (170g) cauliflower, cut into florets
2 oz (55g) mangetout peas or French beans (remove tough strings)
5 tablespoons brown rice vinegar
1 tablespoon shoyu
Chopped parsley to garnish (optional)

American
½ cup carragheen
3 cups water
Pinch of sea salt
2 medium carrots, sliced thinly
1 cup cauliflower, cut into florets
1 cup snow peas or snap beans (remove tough strings)
5 tablespoons brown rice vinegar
1 tablespoon shoyu
Chopped parsley to garnish (optional)

1. Clean and sort out any small stones from the carragheen and rinse quickly several times.
2. Bring the water to the boil with a pinch of sea salt and cook each vegetable separately (removing one before adding the next) for the times indicated in the following order: carrots, 2-3 minutes; cauliflower, 4-5 minutes; peas (or beans), 3-4 minutes. After each vegetable has been boiled, place in a collander and rinse under cold water, then drain.
3. Place the carragheen in the water from the cooked vegetables and soak for 30 minutes.
4. Bring to the boil, reduce the heat and simmer for 1 hour or more until the carragheen has almost dissolved. Stir occasionally to prevent sticking. Add the brown rice vinegar and shoyu and cook for a further 2-3 minutes.
5. Place the vegetables decoratively on a serving dish and pour the carragheen sauce on top. Add chopped parsley to garnish (optional).

Seitan Gravy

Imperial (Metric)	American
¼ oz (7g) carragheen	¼ cup carragheen
1 pint (570ml) water	2½ cups water
Few drops of sesame oil (preferably roasted sesame oil)	Few drops of sesame oil (preferably roasted sesame oil)
2 medium onions, diced	2 medium onions, diced
½ green pepper, finely chopped	½ green pepper, finely chopped
7 oz (200g) seitan wheat gluten, cut in small squares	1 cup seitan wheat meat, cut in small squares
3 tablespoons shoyu	3 tablespoons shoyu

1. Clean and sort out any small stones from the carragheen and rinse quickly several times.
2. Place the carragheen in a pot with water and soak for 30 minutes.
3. Bring to the boil, reduce the heat and simmer for 1 hour or more until the carragheen has almost dissolved. Stir occasionally to prevent sticking.
4. Lightly oil a frying pan and heat. Add the onions and sauté for 5-6 minutes, add the pepper and seitan and sauté for a further 8-10 minutes. Season with the shoyu.
5. Add the carragheen sauce, cover the pot and simmer for 5 minutes.

Note: This gravy is delicious served with stuffed marrow (squash).

Baked Apples with Carragheen Lemon Sauce

Serves 4

Imperial (Metric)	American
¼ oz (7g) carragheen	¼ cup carragheen
1¼ pints (700ml) water	3 cups water
4 medium size apples	4 medium size apples
2 tablespoons raisins	2 tablespoons raisins
Pinch of sea salt	Pinch of sea salt
5 tablespoons barley malt	5 tablespoons barley malt
½ teaspoon cinnamon	½ teaspoon cinnamon
2 tablespoons grated lemon rind	2 tablespoons grated lemon rind

1. Clean and sort out small stones from the carragheen and rinse several times quickly.
2. Place the carragheen in a pot with the water and soak for 30 minutes.
3. Bring to the boil, reduce the heat and simmer for 1 hour or more until the carragheen has almost dissolved. Stir occasionally to prevent sticking.
4. Whilst the carragheen is cooking prepare the apples. With a teaspoon remove the top half of each apple core. In the holes place a pinch of salt and the raisins.
5. Place the filled apples on a baking tray and cook in a moderately hot oven 375°F/190°C (Gas Mark 5) until they are soft.
6. To the cooked carragheen sauce add the barley malt, cinnamon and grated lemon rind and simmer for 5 minutes.
7. Pour this sauce over the baked apples and serve either hot or cold.

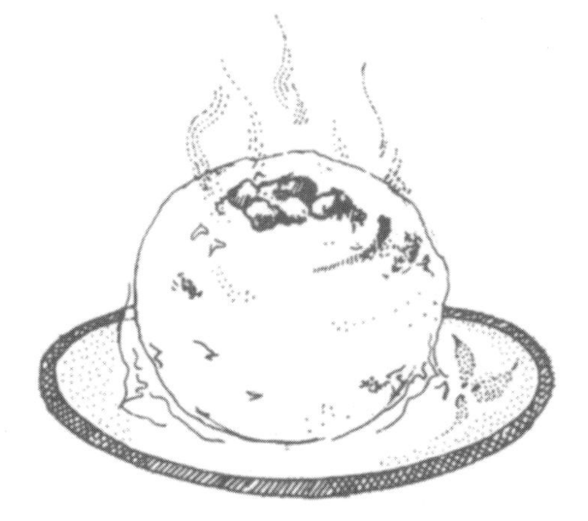

Orange Raisin Sauce

Imperial (Metric)

½ oz (15g) carragheen
1½ pints (850ml) water
9 oz (255g) raisins or sultanas
Pinch of sea salt
2 tablespoons orange rind, grated
Juice from 2 oranges
Barley malt, few teaspoons (optional)
1 oz (30g) chopped roasted hazelnuts

American

½ cup carragheen
3¾ cups water
1½ cups raisins or golden seedless raisins
Pinch of sea salt
2 tablespoons orange rind, grated
Juice from 2 oranges
Barley malt, few teaspoons (optional)
¼ cup chopped roasted filberts

1. Clean and sort out any small stones from the carragheen and rinse quickly several times. Place in a pot with the water and soak for 30 minutes.
2. Bring to the boil, reduce the heat and simmer for ½ hour. Add the raisins, a pinch of sea salt and simmer ½ hour more or until the carragheen has almost dissolved. Stir occasionally to prevent sticking.
3. Add the orange rind and juice.
4. If the sauce is not sweet enough add a few teaspoons of barley malt. Cook for 2-3 minutes.
5. Add the chopped roasted hazelnuts (filberts).
6. Serve this sauce on its own or as a dessert topping, either hot or cold.

Appendix I
Obtaining Sea Vegetables and Other Recipe Ingredients

Sea vegetables in dried form are readily available nowadays in many natural and wholefood stores and increasingly in health food shops. Oriental food stores, especially Japanese, also carry some varieties, although in these stores it is necessary to ascertain the quality first. (Nori and agar-agar are sometimes treated with chemicals.) If you have difficulty obtaining sea vegetables locally, there are mail order houses that can supply you with a full range in a variety of sizes. They can also supply any of the other ingredients mentioned in the recipes. See list on page 134.

For the more adventurous, and to obtain the tastiest supplies, sea vegetables can be harvested fresh around much of the coastline of North West Europe and North America. The best locations are wild areas remote from habitation and industry, where you are sure there is no sewage or industrial effluent discharging into the water. Also these areas will have stronger ocean currents yielding the cleanest, highest quality plants. First do some homework on your chosen area, studying which varieties grow there and learning to identify them with the help of botanical reference books (see *Further Reading*). Then choose your time, ideally at the monthly lowest tide, when the maximum number of species will be uncovered by the water, remembering also that sea vegetables have a growing season and are usually most tender in the spring. Equip yourself with a good cutting knife — you should be looking for live plants, not washed-up debris. After harvesting your sea vegetables they can be sorted and either washed, for cooking and eating fresh, or washed and dried, for storing and using throughout the year.

Mail Order Supplies

Britain

The largest range of sea vegetables in Britain is available from Clearspring, which will supply either wholesale, retail or mail order.

Clearspring Natural Grocer
196 Old Street
London EC1V 9BP
Tel. 01-250 1708

USA

The following companies will mail supplies directly to you or refer you to a distributor in your area:

Eden Foods, Inc.
701 Tecumseh Road
Clinton, MI 49236
Tel. 517-456-7424
Tel. 313-973-9400

Edward and Sons Trading Company
P.O. Box 3150
1091 Lousons Road
Union, NJ 07083
Tel. 201-964-8176

Granum Inc.
2901 N.E. Blakeley Street
Seattle, WA 98105
Tel. 206-525-0051

Mountain Ark Trading Company
120 S. East Street
Fayetteville, AR 72701
Tel. 501-442-7191

Appendix 2
Further Reading

The following books primarily deal with sea vegetables as foods.

Kushi, M. *The Book of Macrobiotics.* Tokyo; Japan Publications Inc., 1977.

Arasaki, S. & T. *Vegetables from the Sea.* Tokyo; Japan Publications Inc., 1983.

Madlener, J. C. *The Sea Vegetable Book.* New York; Clarkson N. Potter, Inc., 1977.

Rhoads, S. A. *Cooking with Sea Vegetables.* Autumn Press, Brookline, MA., USA, 1978.

The following books primarily discuss botanical forms of sea vegetables.

Dickinson, C. I. *British Seaweeds.* The Kew Series. London; Eyre and Spottiswoode, 1963.

Major, A. *The Book of Seaweed.* London; Gordon & Cremonesi, 1977.

Hillson, C. J. *Seaweeds.* Keystone Books, Penn. State U. Press, 1977.

Guberlet, M. L. *Seaweeds at Ebb Tide.* University of Washington Press, 1956.

Appendix 3

Composition of Sea Vegetables Per 100g Edible Portion

	Fibre g	Protein g	Fat g	Carboh. g	Calcium mgs	Iron mgs	Iodine mgs	Phosph. mgs	Potass. mgs	Vit. A iu	Vit. B_1 mgs	Vit. B_2 mgs	Niacin mgs	Vit. C mgs
Nori	4.7	35.0	0.7	39.6	470	23	0.5	510	N.A.	11000	0.25	1.24	10.0	20
Kombu	3.0	7.3	1.1	51.9	800	15	300	150	5800	430	0.08	0.32	1.8	11
Wakame	3.6	12.7	1.5	47.8	1300	13	25	260	6800	140	0.11	0.14	10.0	15
Dulse	1.2	25.0	3.2	44.2	296	150	150	267	8060	N.A.	0.63	0.50	N.A.	30
Hijiki	13.0	5.6	0.8	29.8	1400	29	40	59	14700	150	0.01	0.20	4.6	0
Arame	7.1	12.1	1.3	44.7	1170	12	300	150	3860	50	0.02	0.20	2.6	0
Agar-agar	0	2.3	0.1	74.6	400	5	0.2	8	N.A.	0	0	0	0	0
Carragheen	2.2	9.4	3.2	55.4	885	9	N.A.	157	2844	N.A.	N.A.	N.A.	N.A.	N.A.
Spinach	0.6	3.2	0.3	4.3	93	3	Trace	51	470	8100	0.10	0.20	0.6	51
Cows Milk	0	3.5	3.5	4.9	118	Trace	0	93	144	140	0.03	0.17	0.1	1

Sources: U.S.D.A. and Japan Nutritionist Association food tables. N.A. — information not available.

Appendix 4
Common and Botanical Names of Popular Sea Vegetables

COMMON PLANT NAME	COMMON FOOD NAME	BOTANICAL NAME
Nori and Laver Group		
Sea Lettuce, Green Laver (U.K.)		*Ulva lactuca*
Ao-Nori (JAP.)	Green Nori Flakes	*Monostroma latissima*
Asakusa Nori (JAP.)	Sheet Nori, Sushi Nori, Kizami Nori	*Porphyra tenera*
Wild Nori, Purple Laver (U.K.) Sloke (IRE.), Slake (SCT.)	Laverbread (WLS.), Black Butter (ENG.)	*Porphyra umbilicalis*
Fu-Nori (JAP.)	Purple Leaf Nori	*Gloiopeltis furcata*
Kombu and Kelp Group		
Ma-Kombu, Ne-Kombu etc. (JAP.)	Kombu, Natto Kombu, Tororo Kombu etc. (JAP.)	*Laminaria japonica*
Sugar Wrack, Poor Man's Weatherglass (U.K.)	Sweet Kombu	*Laminaria saccharina*
Bladderwrack, Sea Wrack (ENG.) Pigweed (SCT.)		*Fucus vesiculosus*
(Sea) Tangle, Oarweed, Tangleweed, Sea Girdle (U.K.), Finger Kombu (USA)		*Laminaria digitata*

Other Brown Algae

Wakame (JAP.)	Wakame, Ita Wakame etc. (JAP.)	*Undaria pinnatifida*
Mekabu (JAP.)	'root' Wakame	sporophylls of *U. pinnatifida*
Dabberlocks, Brown Ribweed (ENG.), Murlins (IRE.), Henware (SCT.), Wing Kelp (USA)	Alaria	*Alaria esculenta*
Hijiki (Hiziki) (JAP.)		*Hizikia fusiforme*
Arame (JAP.), Sea Oak, Southern Sea Palm (USA)		*Eisenia bicyclis*

Red Algae

Dulse, Dillisk, etc.		*Palmaria (Rhodymenia) palmata*
Agar-Agar, Tengusa (JAP.)	Kanten (JAP.), Agar flakes, bars & powder.	*Gelidium sp.*
Carragheen, Irish Moss, Dorset Moss, Iberian Moss.		*Chondrus crispus*

Abbreviations — (JAP.) - Japan, (ENG.) - England, (IRE.) - Ireland, (SCT.) - Scotland, (WLS.) - Wales.

Index